# POCKET
# SURGERY

William R. Wrightson, MD
Resident in Surgery
University of Louisville
Louisville, Kentucky

D1521397

**Blackwell**
**Science**

# Blackwell Science

© 2002 by Blackwell Science, Inc.

*Editorial Offices:*
Commerce Place, 350 Main Street, Malden,
Massachusetts 02148, USA
Osney Mead, Oxford OX2 0EL, England
25 John Street, London WC1N 2BS, England
23 Ainslie Place, Edinburgh EH3 6AJ, Scotland
54 University Street, Carlton, Victoria 3053, Australia

*Other Editorial Offices:*
Blackwell Wissenschafts-Verlag GmbH, Kurfürstendamm 57, 10707 Berlin, Germany
Blackwell Science KK, MG Kodenmacho Building, 7-10 Kodenmacho
    Nihombashi, Chuo-ku, Tokyo 104, Japan
Iowa State University Press, A Blackwell Science Company, 2121 S. State Avenue,
    Ames, Iowa 50014-8300, USA

*Distributors:*

*The Americas*
    Blackwell Publishing
    c/o AIDC
    P.O. Box 20
    50 Winter Sport Lane
    Williston, VT 05945-0020
    (Telephone orders: 800-216-2522;
    fax orders: 802-864-7626)

*Australia*
    Blackwell Science Pty, Ltd.
    54 University Street
    Carlton, Victoria 3053
    (Telephone orders: 03-9347-0300;
    fax orders: 03-9349-3016)

*Outside The Americas and Australia*
    Blackwell Science, Ltd.
    c/o Marston Book Services, Ltd.
    P.O. Box 269
    Abingdon
    Oxon OX14 4YN
    England
    (Telephone orders: 44-01235-465500;
    fax orders: 44-01235-465555)

Acquisitions: Beverly Copland
Development: Angela Gagliano
Production: Irene Herlihy
Manufacturing: Lisa Flanagan
Marketing Manager: Toni Fournier
Cover design by Gary Ragaglia
Interior design by Gallagher
Typeset by Gallagher
Printed and bound by DS Graphics

Printed in the United States of America
01 02 03 04   5 4 3 2 1

**Library of Congress Cataloging-in-Publication Data**
Wrightson, William R.
    Pocket surgery / by William R. Wrightson.
        p. ;   cm.
    ISBN 0-632-04615-5 (pbk.)
    1. Surgery—Handbooks, manuals, etc.
    [DNLM: 1. Surgery—Handbooks. 2. Internship and Residency—Handbooks.
    3. Surgical Procedures, Operative—Handbooks. WO 39 W954p 2002] I. Title.
    RD37.2 .W75 2002
    617--dc21                                                    2001002988

# Contents

# Foreword

*Pocket Surgery* is indeed the brainchild of one of our most innovative medical students and resident surgeons, Dr. William R. Wrightson. Every good training program often has nuggets hidden within it of individuals who plumb the depths of understanding for certain detailed aspects of being a good house officer, and others who take those depths and build them into a reliable and broadly applicable understanding of a field that can be shared with their successors on the service. In this case, I believe that this book is a conscientious effort on the part of Dr. Wrightson to examine both the depth of surgery as a whole and to develop an approach to each of the scenarios that relates to student and junior house officer consideration.

We are in a scenario now in which the abbreviated exposure to surgery for undergraduate medical students is the norm and is perhaps becoming even briefer. This is especially difficult since surgery remains one of the four therapeutic options for all human disease and, in my opinion, one that often provides total cure, whether the illness be something as complex as malignant melanoma or something as disturbing as low back pain. As students find their surgical exposure more and more compacted, the need for educational guides such as this specific book seems to grow greater and greater. It is patently impossible to take on the substance of a major surgical text, and many of the shorter efforts have not kept pace with the expansion of surgical concepts and technology.

The future of surgery will be dominated by the kinds of technical advances that have characterized the past decade. The proper projection is that the pace of these advances will be evermore rapid and will evermore involve new uses of computer technology, the Internet, and robotic activity. One must be fully cognizant of this broad and extraordinarily exciting "Star Wars" view of the future of surgery, but this is a hard concept to convey to the student who needs to walk into a clinic tomorrow with some insight and understanding of how to begin the evaluation of a breast lump or abdominal pain.

*Pocket Surgery* is a great beginning for students, because it provides not only educational surgery at the basic level, but, as these students become the next practitioners of medicine, it will also be something that the patients of these doctors will appreciate for the next few decades.

Hiram C. Polk Jr., MD

Ben A. Reid, Professor and Chairman
Department of Surgery
University of Louisville School of Medicine
Louisville, Kentucky

# Preface

While on their surgical rotations, medical students are constantly subjected to quizzing throughout the day. A well-prepared medical student must be ready to respond with the essential facts for each situation. This creates a vital need for a quick-reference guide to use during both rotations and the surgical internship. *Pocket Surgery* provides you with an opportunity to gain insight into basic surgical principles and daily routine. Written specifically for medical students and interns, *Pocket Surgery* brings together the most needed and asked surgical information into a convenient pocket-sized reference. Its unique features enhance understanding and general surgical training.

*Pocket Surgery* offers the advice and information you'll need to make it through your surgical clerkship and internship. The comprehensive outline format ensures that any student using *Pocket Surgery* will find the answers to the surgical questions encountered. This book is not designed to be a reference textbook. However, it will provide the most crucial surgical information immediately. *Pocket Surgery* is the medical student's and intern's survival guide, offering concise, readable, and functional information on the most common topics discussed on rounds and on written and oral exams.

William Wrightson, MD, found a need for just such a book during his surgical rotation. Then as an intern, he again needed this content. When he was unable to find a concise handbook giving him the resources he needed to be prepared for daily quizzing, Dr. Wrightson decided to write this pocket guide to prepare future surgical interns for basic surgical principles and to advise how to handle the daily routine.

Designed to be readily accessible, *Pocket Surgery* is written in an outline structure to streamline information, while providing a readable information base. Featuring "Fact Boxes" that offer valuable information at a glance, this book aims to provide quick answers to common questions, leaving you prepared and knowledgeable. This unique manual for surgical rotation and internship fulfills the need for a handbook for quick reference while on the wards and doubles as an oral and written exam review tool.

We at Blackwell provide this new resource for your surgical rotations and internships and hope that *Pocket Surgery* will become your surgical survival guide!

## Acknowledgments

I would like to thank my wife, Svetlana, for her support and understanding; Hiram C. Polk, Jr., MD, and Susan Galandiuk, MD, for the opportunity to achieve and discover; Mary B. Carter, MD, PhD, for professional advice and encouragement; and Margaret Abby, Vicky Hadley, Shirley Cook, Judy Slaughter, and Debbie Shaut for technical assistance.

WRW

**Notice:** The indications and dosages of all drugs in this book have been recommended in the medical literature and conform to the practices of the general community. The medications described and treatment prescriptions suggested do not necessarily have specific approval by the Food and Drug Administration for use in the diseases and dosages for which they are recommended. The package insert for each drug should be consulted for use and dosage as approved by the FDA. Because standards for usage change, it is advisable to keep abreast of revised recommendations, particularly those concerning new drugs.

# Introduction

Surgery, as a science and an art, is a formidable undertaking for the medical student and even more so for the surgery intern. Surgery is the integration of many medical disciplines and in many respects is the last stand of the true general physician. This text is designed to facilitate and guide you through your surgical rotations.

There are certain rules that the student and intern should be aware of for the wards and oral exams. Following these simple guidelines will help you to do well and have a more enjoyable surgical experience.

## Ward Commandments

1. Be enthusiastic.
2. Be early—start rounding well before your resident (first to arrive and last to leave).
3. Stay on top of lab results and radiology results.
4. Don't complain. (Sleep is for wimps, eating is a waste of time, tired is not a word).
5. "Yes Sir/Ma'am" and "No Sir/Ma'am" are generally the only words that need to be spoken to attendings and chief residents.
6. Write everything down; make *To Do* lists.
7. Never, *NEVER* lie—if you missed something or don't know the lab value . . . fess up.
8. Don't quarrel with the nursing staff. They can hurt you much more than you can hurt them.
9. Follow the chain of command, and always try to make your upper levels look good (i.e., if they are happy, you will be too).
10. Introduce yourself to attendings when you scrub in on cases.
11. Dress appropriately in a clean, professional manner. In general, scrubs are for the OR only.

**Oral Exams**

1. Be prepared.
2. State your answers with confidence.
3. Practice out loud using appropriate terminology (esophagogastroduodenoscopy rather than EGD).
4. When preparing for the exam it is useful to think in terms of the following categories and conduct the exam in the same way.
   - Complete history and physical
   - Simple labs
   - Radiology
   - Diagnostic tests, biopsy
   - Diagnosis
   - Treatment options
   - Follow-up
5. Always go from least expensive/invasive to most expensive/ invasive when ordering diagnostic studies.
6. CT scan is NEVER the correct *first* thing to order.
7. In all cancer cases, once you have a tissue diagnosis, you need to *stage* the patient. In general think of this as a single word: boneliverlungbrain. In other words, most cancers will met to:
   - Bone (PE, bone scan)
   - Liver (LFTs, CT)
   - Lung (CXR)
   - Brain (PE, CT)
8. If you do not have a clue what the answer is, sometimes it is best to say, "I do not know the answer." Remember the most basic statement in science, the beginning of wisdom, is "I do not know."
9. Remember your trauma ABCs (**A**irway, **B**reathing, **C**irculation).

# 1

# Basic Orders: Admit, Post-Op, Pre-Op, Discharge

Surgical orders should include maintenance and care of all tubes, drains, and wounds (Nursing), as well as pain management, antibiotics (Medications), and morning labs (Lab) as needed. Remember to date and time *all* orders. Below are outlines of typical orders.

### Admit/Post-Op Orders

Admission orders are written for any patient entering the hospital or when transferring a patient from one unit to the next. Post-op orders are written after any operation or procedure is performed.

*Date, Time*—

*Admit*—To recovery room (RR), then to ICU/TCU/floor; include name of the surgical service and attending surgeon.

*Computer*—Please place on computer list ###### (for hospitals with computerized census keeping).

*Diagnosis*—List patient's admitting diagnosis or indication for surgery; list the surgical procedure performed if writing post-op orders.

*Condition*—Good, fair, stable, guarded, serious, or critical

*Vitals*—Specify frequency: per shift, routine, q4h, q1h × 4 hours, then q4h, etc.

*Activity*—Bed rest, log roll only, out of bed (OOB), to chair qid, ambulate qid, etc.

*IVF*—Typical maintenance IVF: D5 1/2 NS + 20 mEq KCl per liter (use the 4/2/1 rule to calculate maintenance rate, *see Fluids and Electrolytes*); typical post-op fluids: D5 Lactated Ringer's (LR) at 1.5–2 times maintenance.

*I/O*—Specify when intake and output (I/O) should be recorded (q4h, per shift, routine, etc.) and specify if strict.

*Medications*—Pain meds (patient-controlled analgesia [PCA] morphine or meperidine [Demerol]), nausea meds (promethazine [Phenergan]), acid control (famotidine [Pepcid]), antibiotics, home meds.

*Diet*—NPO strict, NPO except for meds with sips $H_2O$, NPO except for ice chips, clear liquids, full liquids, dental soft, regular diet, or advance diet as tolerated.

*Allergies*—List any medical, environmental, or food allergies.

*Oxygen*—Only if required (e.g., chronic obstructive pulmonary disease [COPD]), usually is 2–4 L nasal cannula (NC) if patient is to go to the floor.

*Drains/Catheters*—Name all tubes and drains, and indicate how maintained, output measurement frequency, type of suction (to gravity, to bulb, to low wall suction [LWS], etc.). For example:

- *Foley*—To gravity at bedside, measure urine output q1 hour, q4h, or q shift
- *Nasogastric Tube (NGT)*—To LWS, irrigate q4h with 50 mL tap water to maintain patent; record output q shift
- *Jackson Pratt (JP)*—To bulb suction, measure output q4h and discard
- *Chest Tube*—To –20 cm LWS, record output q shift

*DVT Prophylaxis*—Compression stockings (TED hose), sequential compression device (SCD), heparin 5000 U sq qd, low-molecular-weight heparin (Lovenox 30 mg sq bid).

*Labs*—Only order labs that will affect the care of the patient. There are no routine labs!

**Pre-Op Orders**

Pre-Op orders include basic information to facilitate transition from the floor (or holding area) to the operating room.

*Date, Time*—

*Diet*—NPO after midnight except for meds with sips $H_2O$.

*Medications*—Antibiotics (e.g., cefazolin [Kefzol] 1g IV on call to OR [OCTOR]), steroids, sleeping meds (to be administered only after consent has been signed), bowel prep.

*Labs*—CBC, BMP, PT/PTT, urinalysis (UA), type and cross (T&C).

*Studies*—Chest x-ray (CXR), electrocardiogram (ECG).

*Consent*—Explain the procedure, risks, and benefits to the patient; insure that the consent form is signed and on the chart for the appropriate procedure.

*Other*—Stop heparin drip OCTOR or within 2 hours of OR time.

---

**FACT BOX 1**

Kefzol® has the longest $t_{1/2}$ of all the first generation cephalosporins, making it a good choice as a prophylactic antibiotic.

---

**Discharge Orders**

*Date, Time*—

*Discharge*—To home, rehab center, nursing home, etc.

*Meds*—Pain meds, antibiotics, iron, Coumadin, resume home meds, etc.

*Diet*—Regular, include any restrictions such as low sodium or high protein.

*Activity*—If post-op, activity usually restricted with no lifting >10 lbs., no tub baths, no swimming, no driving while on pain meds, etc. List work or school restrictions.

*Self-Care*—Dressing changes, wound care, physical therapy, ambulation, daily shower, Sitz bath, etc.

*Follow-Up*—Include appropriate clinic or private office follow-up, labs, or x-rays required at office visit.

*Home Health*—Name of agency and instructions to home health nurse.

*Call MD or Return to ER*—If fever, vomiting, redness around the wound, or discharge from the wound.

# 2

# Notes and Charting

Surgical notes should be concise and accurate. Special mention should be made wherever applicable concerning current antibiotics, drain outputs, wound healing, status of distal pulses, and bowel function. Notes, like orders, should have the date and time documented. Below are outlines of typical notes.

## Preoperative Note

The pre-op notes are a pre-op checklist that is usually performed the night before surgery to identify any problems and insure patient is ready for the OR in morning

*Date, Time—*

*Pre-Op Diagnosis—*e.g., peripheral vascular disease.

*Procedure Planned—*e.g., femoral-popliteal bypass.

*Surgeon(s)—*List attending surgeon and chief resident.

*Anesthesia Planned—*Local, regional, epidural, spinal, or general endotracheal anesthesia (GETA).

*Pre-Op Labs—*Document CBC, BMP, PT/PTT, and correct any problems. Document UA results.

*Blood—*Call the blood bank; confirm that the patient is typed and crossed for *x* units.

*Pre-Op Studies—*Document results of CXR, ECG.

*Consent—*Document whether the consent is signed and on chart.

*Major Medical Problems—*Cardiovascular (CV), respiratory, renal, methicillin-resistant *aureus* (MRSA), human immunodeficiency virus (HIV).

*Medications*—Document whether home meds, bowel prep, sleeping med, if consent signed, and antibiotic IV OCTOR are ordered.

*Diet*—Document whether NPO after midnight except when meds with sips of $H_2O$ are ordered.

*Other*—Stop heparin drip OCTOR. Make sure patients are off any blood thinners (Coumadin, ASA, Plavix).

## Brief Op Report

Written in the OR following the procedure.

*Date/Time*—

*Pre-Op Diagnosis*—e.g., appendicitis.

*Post-Op Diagnosis*—e.g., appendicitis with perforation.

*Procedure(s) Performed*—e.g., appendectomy.

*Surgeons*—Attending, first assistant, second assistant.

*Op Findings*—Any significant findings (tumor, perforation, necrotic bowel, inflamed appendix, pus, blood, etc.).

*Anesthesia*—GETA, regional, spinal, epidural, or local.

*Estimated Blood Loss (EBL)*—Obtain this information from the anesthesiologist.

*Fluids*—From the anesthesiologist (e.g., 2500 mL crystalloid, 2 units packed RBCs, 500 mL colloid).

*Specimens*—Include cultures, pieces of tissue, organs removed, limbs removed, and foreign bodies of forensic interest such as bullets or knife blades.

*Drains*—Type and location (good idea to draw a diagram in the chart if two or more drains placed).

*Complications*—List any complications (ask the attending surgeon first).

*Disposition*—To RR/ICU/TCU in good, stable, guarded, or critical condition.

## Night of Surgery

The purpose of this note is to identify any emerging problems and prevent disasters. The most important findings to document are level of consciousness (recovery from anesthesia), pain control, and urine output (degree of resuscitation).

*Date/Time*—

*Procedure*—Status post (S/P) (name of procedure).

*Level of Consciousness*—Alert, oriented, somnolent, lethargic, nonresponsive.

*Pain Control*—Adequate, poor, excessive reliance, etc.

*Vitals*—Temp, heart rate (HR), blood pressure (BP), respiratory rate (RR). If Swan-Ganz monitor, record cardiac output (CO), cardiac index (CI), pulmonary capillary wedge pressure (PCWP).

*UOP*—Record UOP since surgery. Optimal output is >30 mL/hour for adults, 1 mL/kg/h for children, 2 mL/kg/h for infants.

*Physical Exam*—Breath sounds bilaterally, presence or absence of pulses, etc.

*Wound*—Record whether dressing in place and note if dry or if serosanguineous discharge, etc.

*Labs*—Document results of post-op labs including hemoglobin and hematocrit (H&H), coagulation studies, blood gases, and basic chemistries.

*Assessment*—List problems, document whether hemodynamically stable, satisfactory progress or not.

*Plan*—List strategy to address all problems.

## Daily Progress Note

Each patient will require a directed exam daily focusing on his or her disease process and surgery performed. Below is an example of a daily progress note in the general SOAP format with surgical focus.

### Opening

- Date and time of day
- Hospital day, postoperative day, or postinjury day number
- Antibiotics and day number (e.g., cefazolin [Kefzol], Day 2)

### Subjective

- Complaints or concerns volunteered by patient
- Document also flatus, bowel movement (BM), pain control, activity, diet, nausea, vomiting

### Objective

- Vitals ($T_{max}/T_{current}$, HR, RR, BP)
- UOP by shift
- Drain outputs by shift
- Directed exam, focusing on:
  - Incision for signs of infection (SOI), tenderness, discharge, erythema
  - Distal pulses
  - Bowel sounds
  - Lungs for assessment of pulmonary care
- Labs

### Assessment

- Address any problems or complaints

### Plan

- Eliminate any tubes or drains that are no longer necessary.
- Advance diet as appropriate.
- Order diagnostic studies or labs that are pertinent.
- Change medications as needed (e.g., IV to po).
- Taper pain control.
- Increase ambulation as appropriate.
- Teach patient or patient's family wound care.

Goal is to get the patient well and to a satisfactory status for discharge (D/C).

# 3

# Wounds and Dressings

**Wound Healing**

Inflammation 0–4 days
Epithelialization 1–2 days
Proliferation (fibroplasia) 2–20 days
Contraction/remodeling (4–6 weeks)
  • Wounds regain 50% of tensile strength at 4 weeks and 70% at 8 weeks.
  • Sutures and staples are usually removed 5–7 days postop for most surgical wounds. Some wounds need a full 14 days before suture or staple removal. Wounds on face 5 days, trunk 7–10 days, extremities as long as 14 days secondary to mechanical stresses.

## *Types of Healing*

*Primary Intention*—Wound edges are surgically re-approximated soon after incision/laceration occurs, usually within 4–6 hours.
*Secondary Intention*—Wound edges are left open and dressing changes are performed three times a day (tid). Wound heals by granulation, contraction, and epithelialization over a period of weeks. Used for grossly contaminated wounds.
*Delayed Primary Closure*—Wound edges are initially left open and dressing changes are performed tid. After 2–5 days, granulation tissue forms and wound edges are surgically re-approximated under sterile conditions.

## Types of Dressings

*Surgical*—If wound is closed in the OR, dry gauze is applied. Remove gauze dressing 24–48 hours postop. *Exceptions:* Contaminated wounds are not closed in the OR. In this case, remove dressing 12–24 hours postop and begin wet to dry dressing changes q6–8h.

---

FACT BOX **2**

Remove dressings postop day 1–2 because wound has epithelialized.

---

**TABLE 3.1**
**Types of Dressings**

| Occlusive Dressings | Type | Uses |
| --- | --- | --- |
| Adaptic® | Moisturizing and antibacterial Nonadherent | Used for burns, grafts |
| Scarlet Red | Promotes re-epithelialization | Used for burns, donor sites |
| Op-Site® Tegaderm® (transparent dressing) | Occlusive, impermeable to bacteria and water | Cover central line sites, skin donor sites, small incisions |
| Duoderm® (hydrocolloid dressing) | Hydrocolloid, absorptive, promotes granulation and re-epithelialization | Sacral decubitus ulcers, skin ulceration |

*Wet to Dry Dressings*—Wound is packed with a slightly damp piece of sterile gauze and covered with dry gauze.

• Provides a micro-debridement of the wound when the dressing is changed.
• Dressing changes are usually twice a day (bid), tid, or four times a day (qid).
• Solutions used to moisten the deep layer of sterile gauze include normal saline and dilute hypochlorite (Dakins).

### *Dressing Solutions and Ointments*

- Normal Saline—Used for clean wounds with good granulation tissue
- 0.5% Silver Nitrate ($AgNO_3$)—Antimicrobial, often used for burn wounds
- Dakins (hypochlorite solution) 1/8 strength—Used for mildly contaminated wounds, is antimicrobial, should not deter wound healing
- Dakins 1/4 strength—For grossly contaminated wounds, is antimicrobial, may interfere with wound healing
- Povidone-Iodine (Betadine)—Antimicrobial, used for grossly contaminated wounds and gangrenous digits, interferes with wound healing
- Silver Sulfadiazine (Silvadene)—Used for burns, venous stasis ulcers, diabetic foot ulcers
- Mefamide (Sulfamylon)—Used for burns usually

### *Complications of Dressing Solutions and Ointments*

- Silver Sulfadiazine (Silvadene)—Leukopenia
- Silver Nitrate—Hyponatremia, hypochloremia
- Mafenide (Sulfamylon)—Painful application, metabolic acidosis (carbonic anhydrase inhibitor)

### *Other Agents Used in Wound Healing*

*Collagenase*—Useful as enzymatic debridement in the treatment of chronic or acute wounds. Commonly combined with an antimicrobial ointment

*Platelet-Derived Growth Factor (PDGF)*—Promotes chemotaxis and proliferation of inflammatory cells and collagenase production

*Transforming Growth Factor Beta (TGF-β)*—Promotes fibrosis and proliferation of inflammatory cells

*Epidermal Growth Factor (EGF)*—Promotes proliferation and chemotaxis of inflammatory cells

*Zinc* (220 mg PO qd)—Promotes wound healing

### *Factors That Impair Wound Healing*

- Increased age
- Malnutrition
- Exogenous steroids (vitamin A 10,000 IU helps to counter this effect)
- Foreign body
- Diminished blood supply
- Immunocompromise
- Anemia
- Diabetes
- Radiation therapy
- Infection, sepsis
- Smoking

# 4

# Drains and Tubes

## Overview

In general, drains decrease seroma formation and dead space that can lead to impaired wound healing or abscess formation. Drains in the peritoneal cavity have limited effectiveness in that they are quickly surrounded by omentum, which effectively closes the drain tract.

Drains are monitored either hourly or daily for output. For most drains, it is expected that output should decrease with time. Drains should be removed when they no longer serve a function, i.e., minimal fluid being drained (<20 mL per day). Continued drainage beyond the expected time interval suggests a complication such as hemorrhage, infection, or fistula formation. These require further workup.

Immediately postop, fluid may be serosanguineous (blood tinged). Otherwise, the color of drain fluid is usually straw-colored (serous). Drains in the biliary tree accumulate a deep green or golden-colored fluid (bile) and will form bubbles or have a sudsy appearance when shaken. Chylothorax drainage is white and creamy.

## *Drain Types*

*Closed-Suction Drains*—Have a significantly lower infection rate than open drain systems. Examples of closed-suction drains include Jackson-Pratt (JP), chest tubes, Hemovac (HV).

*Open Drains*—Prone to infection because they allow an open conduit for bacterial migration into the wound. These drains are used for contaminated wounds (abscess drainage) and are slowly retracted to allow for healing from the inside out. Examples include Penrose and Davol sump drains.

**Chest Tube** (see Appendix for placement)

Used for decompression of the pleural space (space between the lung and chest wall). Usually placed on $-20$ cm $H_2O$ suction (though in some cases suction can be as much as $-60$ cm $H_2O$).

### *Indications for Chest Tube*

- Pneumothorax
- Flail chest
- Hemothorax
- Hydrothorax
- Chylothorax
- Pleural effusion
- Post thoracotomy
- Prophylactically if patient on ventilator with high peak inspiratory pressures or high positive end expiratory pressure (PEEP) (>20 cm $H_2O$)

### *Air Leak*

Chest tubes are removed only when there is no air leak. Monitor for air leaks daily by observing bubbles in Pleurevac system. This can be done in many ways:

- Clamp off suction and slowly release, watching for air bubbles as suction returns.
- Request that the patient cough. Increased intrathoracic pressure will produce air bubbles in the Pleurevac if an air leak is present.

NOTE: To check if there is an air leak outside the chest wall, *temporarily* clamp the chest tube as it leaves the chest. Bubbles indicate an air leak in the system.

### Chest Tube Removal

Remove the dressing and cut the retention suture that secures the chest tube. Place a Vaseline-impregnated gauze and several 4 × 4s over the exit site. Go ahead and place tape over this gauze to secure it into position (this will make it much easier to secure once the tube is out). Instruct the patient to take a deep breath and then Valsalva (bear down like having a bowel movement). The increased positive pressure will limit the chances of air entering the thorax. Remove the chest tube with one rapid movement. Secure the dressing with wide silk tape to form an occlusive seal. Always get a chest x-ray after removing a chest tube to assess for pneumothorax. Leave dressing in place for 48 hours.

### Special Considerations

*Pneumothorax*—Chest tube remains on suction until air leak is resolved. Once there is no air leak, take tube off wall suction but leave on water seal for 24 hours. Obtain a CXR after 24 hours. Remove chest tube if no pneumothorax. Repeat CXR after pulling tube to check for recurrence of pneumothorax.

*Hemothorax*—In the trauma setting, if initial blood output is >1000 mL, or if bleeding persists at a rate of >200 mL/hour, the patient needs an exploratory thoracotomy.

*Pleural Effusion*—Remove chest tube when drainage has slowed to less than 100 mL in 24 hours.

*Cardiothoracic Procedures*—Mediastinal tubes should be removed off suction within 24 hours postop. Pleural tubes are usually removed while on suction. Total drainage from pleural tubes should be less than 140 mL/8 h before removing.

### Foley Catheter

A Foley catheter may have as many as three lumens (first lumen to drain urine, second lumen to inflate balloon, third lumen [optional] to irrigate bladder). NOTE: Never use saline to inflate the balloon, as salt crystals may prevent deflation and make catheter difficult to remove.

### *Indications for Placement*

- Monitor hourly urine output (strong correlation to volume status, i.e., "the poor man's Swan")
- Provide bladder drainage and decompression after trauma or bladder surgery
- Irrigate bladder with antimicrobial or antifungal medications

---

**FACT BOX 3**

The Foley catheter is frequently referred to as the "poor man's Swan" in that it is an easy way to assess resuscitation and volume status.

---

### *Indications for Removal*

- Patient is ambulatory.
- Patient does not need precise volume status monitoring.
- Bladder has healed.

### *Special Considerations*

- If patient has sudden decrease in urine output, always irrigate the catheter with 50 mL NS to assess for clot or obstruction. If still in doubt whether catheter is functioning properly, remove and re-insert a new Foley catheter.
- Patients with a documented UTI and a Foley frequently have colonization of the catheter. These patients may benefit from changing the Foley catheter and rechecking the urinalysis.

### Nasogastric Tube

Used mainly for gastric decompression to prevent aspiration of gastric contents. Irrigate tube with 30–50 mL tap water or normal saline (NS) q shift to keep patent. NG tubes are sump drains, meaning they have an air port to provide continuous air flow through the drain. The sump must be functioning; otherwise, the NG tube serves to stent the lower esophageal sphincter (LES) open, increasing risk of aspiration.

### Indications for Placement

- Ileus
- Bowel obstruction
- Unretractable nausea and vomiting
- Postgastrointestinal (GI) or -biliary procedures
- Postsplenectomy

### Indications for Removal

- Decreased drainage
- Return of bowel function
- Conscious and cooperative patient
- Three to five days postsplenectomy
- Seven days post–bowel anastomosis
- When the attending surgeon says

---

**FACT BOX 4**

In postsplenectomy patients the NG serves to keep the stomach decompressed, decreasing the chances of a blowout of ligated short gastric vessels.

---

## GI and Feeding Tubes

*Dobhoff Tube*—Commonly used feeding tube. Placed into stomach via nose. Must obtain abdominal x-ray to confirm placement before beginning feeds. Irrigate with Coca Cola q4–6h to keep patent. This is a temporary means of providing enteral feeds (1–2 weeks).

*Percutaneous Endoscopic Gastrostomy (PEG)*—Placed into stomach through abdominal wall using fiberoptic endoscope. Useful for long-term gastric feeds.

*J Tube*—Placed into the jejunum either surgically or endoscopically. Jejunal feedings are especially useful in patients with pancreatitis or gastric outlet obstruction.

> **FACT BOX 5**
>
> There is no reason to check residuals following J-tube feeds as the tube is beyond the pylorus preventing any risk of aspiration from feeds.

*Sengstaken-Blakemore Tube*—Used for balloon tamponade of bleeding esophageal varices.

*Cecostomy Tube*—Occasionally used to reduce cecal distention, i.e., colonic ileus.

## Vascular and Dialysis Access

*Triple-Lumen Catheter (7F)*—Central venous access for fluids, medications, total parenteral nutrition (TPN), and to draw labs. Appropriate for short term access <1 month.

*Shiley Catheter (12F)*—Large, dual-lumen, central venous catheter. Used for hemodialysis: e.g., acute renal failure, acute overdose, etc. Also excellent for rapid IV fluid infusion (1 L/min).

*Cordis (8.5–9F)*—Large, single-lumen, central venous catheter. Used for rapid fluid infusion (1 L/min). Also needed to place Swan-Ganz catheter through one-way valve.

*Swan-Ganz Catheter*—Useful for hemodynamic monitoring. Tip is positioned in the pulmonary artery.

> **FACT BOX 6**
>
> Swan-Ganz catheters (pulmonary artery catheter [PAC]) provide two fundamental parameters:
> • Volume status
> • Cardiac output or cardiac function

*Infusaport*—Long-term central venous access most commonly used for chemotherapy. Unique in that the entire catheter is under the skin. Must pierce the skin to access the port.

17

*Hickman-Type Catheters*—Indwelling central venous catheter for chemotherapy or TPN.
*Permacath*—Dual-lumen central venous catheter for long-term hemodialysis.
*Tenckhoff Peritoneal Dialysis Catheters*—Used for long-term peritoneal dialysis or drainage of chronic ascites.

---

**FACT BOX 7**

Poisseuille's Law
$$Q = \in P\pi r^4/8l$$

Teaches us that the best catheter for resuscitation is short (small "l") and wide (large "r"). Hence, two large-bore peripheral IV catheters are the gold standard for urgent IV fluid resuscitation.

---

# 5

# Sutures, Needles, and Staples

**Types of Suture Materials**

*Absorbable Suture*

*Chromic Catgut*—Absorbs in 20 days, multifilament. Used in OB/GYN cases and to close tongue lacerations.

*Polyglactin (Vicryl)*—Absorbs in 60 days, most commonly used absorbable suture, good strength knots with 3 throws. Often used for bowel anastomoses and to close skin (subcuticular stitch).

*Polyglycolic Acid (Dexon)*—Absorbs in 60 days, minimal tissue reaction, monofilament.

*Polyglyconate (Maxon)*—Absorbs in 60 days, makes a secure knot, increased strength.

*Polydioxanone (PDS)*—Absorbs in 60 days. Useful in fascial closures.

---

**FACT BOX 8**

Fascial closure is best done by 4 to 1 rule. Use 4 cm of suture for every 1 cm advance in closure.

---

### Nonabsorbable Suture

*Silk Protein Filament*—Good strength, easy to handle, knots with 3 throws. Used to tie off bleeders and for serosal closure in bowel anastomoses.

*Nylon Mono- and Multifilament Forms (Ethilon)*—Commonly used for skin closure. Knots with 6–8 throws.

*Polyester (Ethibond)*—Knots need 5 throws. Often used to secure chest tubes.

*Polypropylene (Proline)*—Used for fascial closure and vascular anastomoses. Knots require 7–10 throws.

*Steel*—Used for sternal closure and delayed primary closure of infected wounds.

### Monofilament Suture

*Advantage*—Less reactive, decreased incidence of infection

*Disadvantage*—Difficult knotting. Must tie 7 or more throws in each knot to secure

*Examples*—Nylon mono- and multifilament forms (Ethilon), polypropylene (Proline)

### Multifilament or Braided Suture

*Advantage*—Easier to handle with more secure knot properties. Knots require only 3–4 throws.

*Disadvantage*—More prone to infection.

*Examples*—Silk, polyglactin (Vicryl).

### Needles

*Cutting*—For tissues such as skin and dermis (Caution: will cut suture)

*Tapered*—For soft vulnerable tissue such as intestine, liver, spleen, and blood vessels

*Blunt*—For friable tissues or for cannulating

### Staples

*Skin Stapler*—Places stainless steel staples through two edges of an incision, one staple at a time. Must evert skin edges prior to application to minimize scar formation and maximize wound healing.

*TA (transverse anastomosis)*—Places a double row of linear everting staggered staples (row may be 30, 55, 90 mm long).

*GIA (gastrointestinal anastomosis)*—Places two double rows of staggered staples and divides the tissues between. Commonly used for bowel resection.

*EEA (end-to-end anastomosis)*—Places a 360E circumferential double row of staggered staples and trims the ends of the bowel. Used to make end-to-end or end-to-side intestinal anastomosis with serosal apposition.

*LDS (ligating-dividing stapler)*—Places two metal clips on either side of a dividing blade. Used to take down omentum or mesentery.

# 6

# Fluids and Electrolytes

## Total Body Water (TBW)

Makes up 60% of total body weight
- TBW = weight in kg $\times$ 0.60 (i.e., 70 kg $\times$ 0.6 = 42 L)
- 2/3 is intracellular (28 L)
- 1/3 is extracellular (14 L)

---

**FACT BOX 9**

In general to replace 1 L of intravascular volume, you must give 3 L of crystalloid. This is due to redistribution of the fluid (i.e., 1/3 extracellular and 2/3 intracellular).

---

## Intravascular Volume

Makes up 7% of total body weight, includes plasma plus blood cells
- Intravascular volume = weight in kg $\times$ 0.07 (i.e., 70 kg $\times$ 0.07 = 4.9 L)
- Red blood cell (RBC) volume = intravascular volume $\times$ Hct, (i.e., 4.9 L $\times$ 0.4 = 1.96 L)
- Plasma volume = intravascular volume – RBC volume (i.e., 4.9 liters – 1.96 liters = 2.94 L)

**Estimation of Maintenance Fluids**

For the typical patient is best determined by 4-2-1 rule:
- 4 mL/h × kg body weight for the first 10 kg body weight (max 40 mL/h)
- 2 mL/h × kg body weight for the next 10 kg body weight (max 20 mL/h)
- 1 mL/h each remaining kg body weight
  *Example:* 8-kg baby should get 4 × 8 = 32 mL/h
  *Example:* 70-kg adult should get 40 + 20 + 50 = 110 mL/h

*Other Methods to Estimate Maintenance Fluids (adults only)*

- 60 mL/h plus 1 mL/h for each kg over 20 kg
  *Example:* 70-kg adult should get 60 + 50 = 110 mL/h
- 1.5 × body weight in kg (rough estimate)
  *Example:* 70-kg adult should get 1.5 × 70 = 105 mL/h

**Types of Fluid Replacement**

*Maintenance Fluids*

Usually have sugar in the form of 5% dextrose (D5)
- D5 1/2NS + 20 mEq potassium chloride (KCl) per liter is the *most common* maintenance fluid for adults
- D5 1/4NS + 10 mEq KCl per liter is the *most common* maintenance fluid for children
- D5 lactated Ringer's (LR)
- D5 NS
- Fresh frozen plasma or D5W is satisfactory maintenance fluid for patients with Child's Class B or C cirrhosis. Must avoid all salt administration in these patients. Albumin and purified protein fraction (PPF) are usually dissolved in salt solutions and should be avoided in patients with cirrhosis.

*Resuscitation Fluids: Crystalloids*

Should *not* have dextrose in them. Resuscitation with solutions containing dextrose will cause hyperglycemia and an osmotic diuresis. Rate of resuscitation depends on urgency. Varies from twice maintenance to 1 L/min.

- LR is classically the fluid of choice for resuscitation.
- NS best if patient has renal failure.
- Electrolyte (Normosol) solutions are often used intraop.

---

**FACT BOX 10**

Albumin is osmotically active and draws fluid intravascularly. Albumin (25 g) is osmotically equivalent to 500 cc NS. Good choice for lung resection or cardiac surgery.

---

## Ionic Makeup of Replacement Fluids

*Normal Saline (NS)*

- 154 mEq sodium (Na), 154 mEq chloride (Cl)

*1/2 Normal Saline (NS)*

- 77 mEq Na, 77 mEq Cl

*Lactated Ringer's (LR)*

- 130 mEq Na
- 110 mEq Cl
- 28 mEq lactate
- 4 mEq potassium (K)
- 3 mEq calcium (Ca)

## Hyperkalemia

Increased potassium ($\uparrow K^+$)

*Etiology*—Renal failure, salt substitutes, blood transfusion, anesthetics, other iatrogenic causes

*Symptom*—Weakness, flaccid paralysis, increased deep tendon reflexes (DTR), mental status changes

*ECG*—Peaked T, wide QRS, and no P wave. As $K^+$ approaches, 7–8 mEq get ventricular fibrillation (V-fib)

### *Rapid Treatment*

- Calcium gluconate one amp IV (10 mL of 10% or 1 g).
- Bicarbonate 1 amp IV of 7.5% (44.6 mEq) causes an intracellular $K^+$ shift.
- $D_{50}W$ 1 amp IV push (50 mL) given with 10–15 units regular insulin IV push causes intracellular $K^+$ shift.

### *Slow Treatment*

- Sodium polystyrene sulfonate (Kayexalate) 1 g/kg retention enema q6h

*Long-Term Control for Patients with Renal or Liver Disease*

- Kayexalate 0.5–1 g/kg PO q day (max dose 30–60 g)

---

**FACT BOX 11**

Hemolysis is frequently the cause of a falsely elevated potassium.

---

### Hypokalemia

Decreased potassium ($\downarrow K^+$)

*Etiology*—Diuretics, malnutrition, excessive vomiting, diarrhea, excess aldosterone.

*Symptoms*—Weakness, muscle cramps, tetany, nausea/vomiting/ileus.

*ECG*—T wave dissipates and U wave appears.

---

**FACT BOX 12**

Persistent hypokalemia may be secondary to hypomagnesemia.

---

### Rapid Treatment

- KCl 10–20 mEq in 50 mL NS over 1 hour IV × 4 (known as $K^+$ runs)
- Maximum $K^+$ replacement: 20 mEq/hour IV
- Check magnesium level and treat if low

### Slow Treatment

- KCl 20–40 mEq PO bid to tid (e.g., K-Dur®)

### Hypernatremia

Increased sodium ($\uparrow Na^+$)

*Etiology*—Sweating, burns, renal failure, lack of free water intake, diabetes insipidus (DI).

*Symptoms*—Confusion, stupor, mental status changes, coma, muscle tremors, and seizures. Rarely pulmonary and peripheral edema.

*Calculation of Free Water Deficit*—Serum sodium concentration is a function of TBW by virtue of osmotic effect. The degree of water deficit can be approximated by calculating the degree of Na excess as:

- Water deficit (liters) = (0.6 × body weight kg)*(serum Na – normal Na)/normal Na.

### Treatment

*Hypovolemic Hypernatremia*

- NS IV—Correct the volume deficit first, then administer free water (D5W) to correct hypernatremia.
- DI—dDAVP (desmopressin) 5–20 mg intranasally or 2 μg IV/SQ q12.

*Normovolemic Hypernatremia*

- D5W—Give 1/2 deficit first 24 hours and the full amount within 48 hours.

## Hyponatremia

Decreased sodium ($\downarrow Na^+$)

*Etiology*—Vomiting, diarrhea, renal failure syndrome of inappropriate antidiuretic hormone (SIADH), congestive heart failure, excess free water intake, decreased aldosterone, hypothyroid, nephrotic syndrome, cirrhosis

*Symptoms*—Lethargy, confusion, coma, mental status changes, muscle twitches, seizures, nausea, vomiting, ileus

### *Treatment*

*Volume Depleted (vomiting, diarrhea)*

• NS IV

*Dilutional*

• Restrict fluids that are hypotonic (e.g., water, soda, milk, coffee, tea, lemonade) to 500 mL/8h.
• Demecocycline 300–600 mg PO q12h for chronic SIADH
• 3% NaCl solution if patient symptomatic
• Caution: Correct $Na^+$ slowly (<2 mEq/L/h) and stop when symptoms resolve. Rapid correction can result in cerebral edema or pontine myelinolysis.

## Hypercalcemia

Increased calcium ($\uparrow Ca^{++}$)

*Etiology*—Bony metastases, hyperparathyroidism, milk alkali syndrome

*Symptoms*—Anorexia, nausea, vomiting, polyuria, polydipsia, constipation, abdominal pains and renal colic, fatigue, hypotonia, coma, psychosis

*ECG*—Short QT interval

*Treatment*

• NS IV at 300–400 mL/h
• Furosemide (Lasix7) 40 mg IV (diuresis with NS and furosemide treats most cases)

- Mithramycin 25 mcg/kg IV over 2–3 hours
- Calcitonin 4 IU/kg IM q12h
- Consider hemodialysis

## Hypocalcemia

Decreased calcium ($\downarrow Ca^{++}$)

*Etiology*—Hypoparathyroidism (most common after thyroid/parathyroid surgery), hemodialysis, blood transfusions

*Symptoms*—Peripheral and perioral paresthesias, increased DTR, abdominal pain and cramps, lethargy, seizures

*Chvostek's Sign*—Face twitches with tap on cheek

*Trousseau's Sign*—Carpal spasm with inflation of blood pressure (BP) cuff above systolic pressure for 2–3 minutes

*ECG*—Prolonged QT interval

*Treatment*

- Calcium gluconate 1 amp IV (10 mL of 10% solution)
- Check magnesium (Mg) levels, treat if low (see hypomagnesemia)

*Chronic Treatment*

- Vitamin D plus oral calcium supplementation (e.g., 400 IU PO qd + 1500 mg PO tid)
- If patient is on hemodialysis, phosphate binders (e.g., Amphojel 300–600 mg PO q4–6h)

## Hypermagnesemia

Increased magnesium ($\uparrow Mg$)

*Etiology*—Iatrogenic, total parenteral nutrition (TPN), renal failure

*Symptoms*—Nausea, vomiting, hyporeflexia, weakness, respiratory failure, bradycardia

*Treatment*

- Calcium gluconate 1 g (10 mL of 10% calcium gluconate) IV

## Hypomagnesemia

Decreased magnesium (↓Mg)

*Etiology*—Malnutrition, lack of supplementation while on IV fluids or TPN

*Symptoms*—Same as hypocalcemia

*Treatment*

- Magnesium sulfate 4 g in 500 mL NS or D5W IV over 4 hours daily

# 7

# Blood and Blood Products

**Oxygen Carriers**

*Packed Red Blood Cells (PRBC)*

- Indicated for hemorrhage, low hematocrit (HCT), anemia. Goal to keep hemoglobin (Hgb) >8 g/dL. Elderly patients and those with cardiac disease may benefit with Hgb >10 g/dL.
- 300–350 mL per unit.
- Each unit raises HCT by 3% to 4% and Hgb by 1.0 g/dL.
- Type and crossmatch required.
- Contains no platelets or clotting factors.

*Whole Blood*

- 450 mL per unit
- Deficient in platelets and factors V, VIII, and XI
- Not available in most centers

### TABLE 7.1
### Transfusion Transmitted Disease Incidence

| Transmitted Disease | Incidence of Transmission |
|---|---|
| Hepatitis C | 1:100,000 |
| Hepatitis B | 1:200,000 |
| HIV | 1:450,000 |

FACT BOX **13**

> Despite current popular press and public fear, patients have a fourfold increased risk of contracting hepatitis as compared to HIV following a blood transfusion.

### Complications of Blood Transfusion

- Hemolytic transfusion reaction
- Infectious viral transmission
- Febrile and allergic reactions
- Coagulopathy
- Hypocalcemia, hyperkalemia
- Hypothermia
- Immunosuppression (avoid transfusions in postop cancer patients)
- Increased risk of cancer recurrence

## Coagulation Components

### Platelets

Indications for the administration of platelets include:

1. Thrombocytopenia (platelets <60K/dL) in the face of active bleeding
2. Preoperative thrombocytopenia (goal is to raise platelets to >100K/dL)
3. Severe thrombocytopenia (platelet count <20K/dL, increased risk of spontaneous bleed)

### Platelet Transfusion

- Volume approximately 175 mL per 10 units.
- No crossmatch necessary, ABO and Rh compatibility recommended.
- Order 6–10 units at a time; blood bank will "pool" the units.
- Each unit should raise platelets ~10K.

### *Fresh Frozen Plasma (FFP)*

- Indicated for bleeding in the face of elevated PT/PTT or Coumadin toxicity.
- Contains all coagulation factors, including 200 units of factor VIII per unit.
- No crossmatch required; however, must be ABO compatible.
- Each unit contains 150–200 mL volume.
- Order 4–6 units at a time.

### *Cryoprecipitate*

- Indicated for bleeding in the face of hemophilia A, von Willebrand's disease, low fibrinogen, or after cardiopulmonary bypass (CPB) to correct coagulopathy.
- Each unit contains 80 international units of factor VIII and 150 mg fibrinogen in 15 mL volume.
- Also contains von Willebrand's factor, factor XIII, and fibronectin.
- Order 8–10 units at a time; blood bank will pool the units.
- No crossmatch required, but ABO compatibility is recommended.

### Colloid

### *Albumin*

- 25 g is osmotically equal to 500 mL plasma.
- 5% solution is diluted in 250–500 mL NS for most situations.
- Can give 5% solution undiluted 4 mL/min.
- Contains sodium, is not recommended for patients with cirrhosis.

### *Purified Protein Fraction (PPF)*

- Albumin and 17% globulin
- Contains sodium, not recommended for patients with cirrhosis

### *Hetastarch (Hespan)*

- Artificial colloid

- Exacerbates bleeding disorders and congestive heart failure (CHF)
- Not recommended in the treatment of trauma patients or perioperatively in any patient

### *Crystalloid*

- Volume expansion with lactated Ringer's (LR) most often recommended (see Chapter 6: Fluids and Electrolytes)

## Hemostasis and Coagulation

A careful history is the best way to assess for bleeding problems in a patient. Coagulation studies may be necessary if you are uncertain or to establish a baseline.

Hemostasis is achieved when a blood vessel is ruptured or severed resulting in vascular spasm, formation of platelet plug, blood coagulation, and growth of fibrous tissue into the clot.

### *Platelets*

- Forms platelet plug
- Action inhibited by ASA (cyclooxygenase inhibitor)
- 7-day life span
- Bleeding time to assess for platelet function

---

**FACT BOX 14**

Platelet dysfunction from ASA or uremia can be partially reversed with DDAVP, which stimulates endothelial release of von Willebrand's factor.

---

### *Coagulation Cascade*

*Intrinsic Pathway*

- Factor XII.
- Contact with exposed tissue collagen activates the cascade.
- Measured by partial thromboplastin time (PTT).

*Extrinsic Pathway*

- Factor VII.
- Tissue thromboplastin activates VII and the cascade.
- Measured by the prothrombin time (PT).

---

**FACT BOX 15**

PT measures extrinsic system (PeT).
PTT measures intrinsic system (PiTT).

---

*Final Common Pathway*

- Factors XIII and IX activate factors X and V, which activate prothrombin to thrombin.
- Thrombin then catalyzes the conversion of fibrinogen to fibrin.

### Common Anticoagulants

*Indications for Anticoagulation*

- Deep venous thrombosis (DVT)
- DVT prophylaxis
- Vascular bypass
- Acute arterial thrombosis
- Atrial fibrillation

*Heparin*

- Activates antithrombin III
- Affects the intrinsic pathway
- Monitored by the pTT (factors VIII, IX, XI, and XII)
- Reverses with protamine
- Half-life is 90 minutes

*Coumadin*

- Inhibits vitamin K–dependent enzymes (II, VII, IX, X)
- Inhibits proteins C and S (must have heparin anticoagulation before starting Coumadin)
- Affects the extrinsic pathway

- Monitor by the PT (factors II, V, VII, and X).
- Vitamin K reverses the effect over 24 hours (vitamin K 5–10 mg sq or IV); use FFP for acute reversal.
- Half-life is 48 hours.

---

**FACT BOX 16**

Since Coumadin's $t_{1/2}$ is 48 hours, a change in dose will not take effect for 2 days.

---

# 8

# Nutrition

**Assessment of Caloric Requirements**

A quick estimation of calorie requirement in adults is 35–40 kcal/kg body weight/day with 1 g/kg/day of protein. Surgical patients usually require 2500 calories or more per day. These values will fluctuate based on metabolic demands of the body in stressed conditions. For patients in the intensive care unit (ICU), a metabolic cart may allow for a more accurate assessment of caloric needs. Patients with carbon dioxide ($CO_2$) retention or who are weaning off the ventilator may benefit from decreasing calories from carbohydrates and increasing calories from fat.

**TABLE 8.1**
**Calorie Content of Basic Food Substances**

| | |
|---|---|
| Fat | 9 kcal/g |
| Protein | 4 kcal/g |
| Carbohydrates | 3.4 kcal/g |

**TABLE 8.2**
**Recommended Composition of Dietary Formulae Based on 2500 Calories/Day Diet**

| | Percentage of Total Calories | Calories |
|---|---|---|
| Carbohydrate | 60% | 1500 |
| Protein | 30% | 750 |
| Lipid | 10% | 250 |
| Total | | 2500 |

## Enteral Nutrition

If the gut works, use it. Early enteral feeding has been shown to decrease postoperative complications including infection and sepsis. Dobhoff or nasogastric (NG) tubes suffice for feeding less than 4 weeks. For extended feeding, use a percutaneous feeding tube (e.g., percutaneous endoscopic gastrostomy (PEG), J tube). Standard feeding solutions are 1–2 Cal/mL.

### *Gastric Feeds*

- Start continuous feeding at 25 mL/h full strength.
- Check gastric residuals by aspirating the stomach contents q4h; hold tube feeds for 1 hour if gastric residual is >150 mL.
- If gastric residuals remain elevated (>150 mL), treat with metoclopramide (Reglan) 10 mg via tube q6–8h.
- If gastric residuals are <150 mL, increase rate of feeds by 25 mL/h increments every 8 hours to goal caloric rate.
- Elevate head of bed for all patients receiving gastric tube feedings
- For every increase in tube feeds, reduce IVF accordingly.
- Once patient is tolerating tube feeds without high residuals, change IV medications to elixir form.
- Flush tube q4h with water or Coca-Cola to maintain patency.
- Do not put crushed-up sucralfate (Carafate) down feeding tubes. This will clog the tube.

---

**FACT BOX 17**

Methylene blue added to feeding solution can help identify aspiration. If respiratory secretions are blue tinged, this suggests ongoing aspiration.

---

### *Jejunal Tube Feeds*

- Start continuous feeds at 25 mL/h full strength.
- No need to check residuals.
- Hold feeds if abdominal distention or nausea.
- Increase rate by 10 mL/h until goal.
- For every increase in tube feeds decrease IVFs accordingly.

*Complications of Enteral Feeds*

- Aspiration (decreased incidence of aspiration associated with J-tube feedings).
- Diarrhea.
- Esophagitis.
- Sinusitis (especially for NG tubes).
- Patients pull out NG and Dobhoff tubes, requiring re-insertion and repeat x-ray for confirmation of placement. This is costly and results in decreased nutritional intake.

**Parenteral Nutrition**

*Peripheral Parenteral Nutrition*

- Suffices for nutritional support lasting less than 72 hours.
- TPN solutions of less than 1000 mOsm are recommended to decrease risk of phlebitis.
- Maximum dextrose solution of 10% can be used (greater values will cause sclerosis of the veins).

*Total Parenteral Nutrition (TPN)*

- Central venous catheter is required due to increased similarity of the delivered solution.
- Percutaneous intravenous central catheter (PICC) line with tip in the subclavian vein or superior vena cava is also satisfactory.

**TABLE 8.3**
**Example of Regular Insulin Sliding Scale**

| Blood Glucose | Treatment |
|---|---|
| 0–60 | 1 AMP D50 |
| 61–100 | 1/2 AMP D50 |
| 101–200 | No treatment |
| 201–250 | 3 U reg insulin |
| 251–300 | 6 U reg insulin |
| 301–350 | 9 U reg insulin |
| 351–400 | 12 U reg insulin* |
| 401–450 | 15 U reg insulin* |

*Recheck blood glucose after administration.

- Always stop IVF once TPN starts as total fluid requirement is met with the TPN
- Glucose checks q6h necessary for all patients on TPN regardless of history of diabetes. Control hyperglycemia with regular insulin sliding scale. Once the daily insulin requirements are established, insulin may be added to the TPN solution.

### Typical TPN Solution

*Carbohydrate* (3.4 Cal/g)—Usually as $D_{20}$, can range from $D_{10}$ to $D_{50}$, e.g., $D_{10}$ has 100 g/L dextrose (340 Cal/L).

*Amino Acids*—5% solution typically.

*Lipids*—10% (1 Cal/mL) or 20% (2 Cal/mL) lipid emulsion. Contains essential fatty acids. Typical volume is 250 cc. Lipids are recommended either daily or every other day.

*Medications*—E.g., Pepcid 40 mg, regular insulin 10 U.

*Other Additives*—Including vitamins, minerals, electrolytes, and micronutrients should usually be included.

### Complications

*Line Sepsis* Typically due to *Staph. epidermidis* or *Staph. aureus*. Fungemia may occur in severely immunocompromised patients. Treat by removing the line. May require a course of antibiotics or antifungals if patient remains septic after line removed.

*Gallstones*—Incidence of cholelithiasis and biliary sludge increases with duration of parenteral feeding.

*Hepatic Steatosis*—Results in increased liver enzymes (AST, ALT). Treat by decreasing dose of lipid emulsion.

*Refractory Hyperglycemia*—Treat by reducing concentration of dextrose and increasing insulin added to TPN solution.

---

FACT BOX **18**

Risk of fungal sepsis:
- Treatment with multiple antibiotics
- TPN
- Central line

# 9

# Respiratory Care and Ventilators

The process of acquisition, transport, and utilization of oxygen is called *respiration*. The process of carbon dioxide ($CO_2$) elimination by the lungs is called *ventilation*.

## Pulmonary Function Testing

### Normal Values (Adult)

| TABLE 9.1 | |
|---|---|
| **Pulmonary Function Normal Values** | |
| Tidal volume | 0.5 L (7–12 mL/kg) |
| Functional residual capacity | 2–3 L |
| Vital capacity | 4–5 L |
| FEV1 | 2–3 L |
| FEV1/FVC | >70% |

### Ventilation/Perfusion Ratio

Describes how much a segment of lung is ventilated in relation to its perfusion. The maintenance of normal gas exchange (oxygenation of circulating blood and elimination of $CO_2$) is a function of the ventilation perfusion ratio. Optimal ratio is a value of 1:1.

## Maximizing Ventilation and Perfusion

*Ventilation*—Collapsed alveoli cause a right-to-left shunt, which means blood passes through the lung without becoming oxygenated. Presence of a right-to-left shunt causes increased need for supplemental oxygen ($O_2$). Ventilation can be improved by opening collapsed alveoli, maximizing lung volume. Techniques include:

- PEEP
- Continuous positive airways pressure (CPAP)
- Coughing
- Deep breathing
- Altering patient position: getting the patient out of bed significantly improves respiratory function
  - A change from the supine to upright position corresponds to an increase of approximately 5 to 12 cm $H_2O$ PEEP

*Perfusion*—Can be improved by optimizing oxygen delivery (maximize cardiac output, hemoglobin (Hgb) concentration, saturation ($SaO_2$), and $O_2$ dissociation curve. Techniques include:

- Transfusion: desired Hgb concentration is 8–10 g/dL for young patients, 10–12 g/dL for older patients
- Reverse alkalemia
- Prevent or correct hypothermia
- Hyperventilation is a common cause of alkalemia in patients on ventilators and should be avoided for this reason. Exception: patients with head injury.

## Oxygen Therapy

### Terminology

- Oxygen saturation ($SaO_2$) describes the percent hemoglobin that is complexed to oxygen. $SaO_2$ is measured with a light probe attached to the finger or ear. Goal is to maintain the saturation of Hgb between 88% and 95%.
- Partial pressure of oxygen in arterial blood ($PaO_2$ or $pO_2$) describes the amount of $O_2$ that is dissolved in the serum but is not complexed to hemoglobin. $PaO_2$ is measured gases.

- Increases in the fraction of inspired oxygen ($FiO_2$) usually improve $SaO_2$ and $PaO_2$, except in cases when a right-to-left shunt is responsible for hypoxemia.
- Partial pressure of $CO_2$ ($PaCO_2$ or $pCO_2$) is not affected by changes in oxygen therapy.

### TABLE 9.2
### Rule of Thumb for $O_2$ Saturation Monitors

| $SaO_2$ | $PaO_2$ |
|---------|---------|
| 90% | 60 torr |
| 80% | 50 torr |
| 70% | 40 torr |

### TABLE 9.3
### Supplemental Oxygen

| | |
|---|---|
| Nasal cannula | Each liter of $O_2$ increases the $FiO_2$ by 4% (maximum 6 liters) |
| Face mask with reservoir | 60% $FiO_2$ at 6 liters, 100% $FiO_2$ at 10 liters |
| Venturi mask | Choice of 24%, 28%, 35%, or 40% $FiO_2$ delivery |
| Bag valve mask | Delivers 100% $FiO_2$ at 15 liters (standard resuscitation) |

### $O_2$ Toxicity

- Sustained elevations in $FiO_2$ >60% result in alveolar collapse, inflammatory changes, alveolar neutrophil infiltration, and eventual fibrosis.
- The lowest concentration of inspired $O_2$ that provides an acceptable $PaO_2$ should always be selected.
- Inspired oxygen concentrations <60% are well tolerated for long periods without clinically evident toxicity.

## Indications for Ventilatory Support

### Inadequate Ventilation

- Apnea
- Acute increase in arterial carbon dioxide tension ($pCO_2$ >50 torr)
- Acidosis
- Chest trauma/flail chest
- Mental status change
- Glasgow score 8 or less

### Inadequate Oxygenation

- Acute decrease in oxygen tension ($pO_2$ <60 torr)
- Severe pulmonary edema
- Adult respiratory syndrome (ARDS)
- Chest trauma
- Aspiration
- Inhalational injury
- Sustained tachypnea with RR >30

## Types of Mechanical Ventilators

- Time cycled
- Volume cycled
- Pressure cycled
- High frequency

### Types of Mechanical Ventilation

#### Controlled Mechanical Ventilation (CMV)

- Delivers preset tidal volume and rate
- No spontaneous breaths allowed
- Paralysis and sedation required
- Commonly used for intraoperative ventilation

#### Assist Control (AC)

- Deliver preset tidal volume every time patient initiates breath.
- Patient does none of the "work" of breathing.

- Allows a nonparalyzed patient to remain completely at rest.
- Backup rate of 10 is usually set in case patient does not initiate any breath or is paralyzed.
- Excellent for patients in septic or cardiogenic shock or in ARDS.
- Cannot be used to wean patient.

---

**FACT BOX 19**

AC can lead to respiratory alkalosis if respiratory rates are high.

---

*Intermittent Mandatory Ventilation (IMV)*

- Preset tidal volume and rate.
- If synchronized intermittent mandatory ventilation (*SIMV*), machine breaths are synchronized to the patient's initiation.
- Patient can breathe faster than over the preset rate; machine provides $O_2$ for such spontaneous respirations but no ventilatory force.
- As preset rate is reduced, patient does more and more "work" of breathing.
- Choice mode for weaning off ventilator.

***Pressure Support***

- Delivers gas at a preset pressure when initiated by patient
- Decreases inspiratory work
- Makes weaning difficult

**Mechanical Ventilation**

| TABLE 9.4 Common Initial Ventilator Settings | |
| --- | --- |
| $FiO_2$ | 40–50% (can start with 100%, wean rapidly) |
| Tidal volume | 6–10 mL/kg body weight |
| Ventilatory rate | 10–14 breaths/min |

Note: Check arterial blood gas 30 minutes after initiating mechanical ventilation.

44

| TABLE 9.4 (continued) | |
| --- | --- |
| PEEP | 3–5 cm $H_2O$ standard |
| I/E (inspiratory/expiratory) | 1:3 |
| Pressure support | 10–15 mm $H_2O$ |
| PIP alarm (peak inspiratory pressure) | Goal is to keep PIP <45 cm $H_2O$. Set alarm to "signal" when PIP >35–40. |

*Examples*

- Frail 80-year-old woman who weighs 65 kg: rate 14, volume 650 mL, $FiO_2$ 50%, PEEP 5 cm $H_2O$, pressure support 10.
- 22-year-old male, weight 85 kg, in ARDS: rate 12, volume 900, $FiO_2$ 70%, PEEP 10 cm $H_2O$, pressure support 10.
- Always check an arterial blood gas 30 minutes after initiating mechanical ventilation.

### *Manipulation of the Ventilator*

There are two primary physiologic parameters that the ventilator controls:
- Ventilation
- Oxygenation

*Ventilation*—The process of $CO_2$ elimination by the lungs. Adequacy of ventilation is determined by measuring the $PaCO_2$ (or $pCO_2$) from arterial blood gas. $pCO_2$ can be affected by changes in:
- Respiratory rate (increase in respiratory rate will decrease $pCO_2$)
- Tidal volume (increase in tidal volume will decrease $pCO_2$)
- Goal $pCO_2$ of 40 mm Hg

*Oxygenation*—Correlates with the $pO_2$ and is controlled by:
- $FiO_2$ (increases in $FiO_2$ will increase $pO_2$)
- PEEP (increases in PEEP will increase $pO_2$)
- Goal $pO_2$ of approximately 90 (sats ≥93%) in healthy patients

### Factors That Increase $O_2$ Consumption

- Fever
- Sepsis

- Burn injury
- Overfeeding
- Seizures
- Shivering
- Agitation
- Vigorous respiratory effort (respiratory rate over 20 breaths per minute, use of accessory muscles of respiration, etc.)
- Sedation (Versed 1–2 mg IV q 1 hour) and pharmacologic paralysis (vecuronium bromide [Norcuron] 10 mg IV q1h) valuable in reducing $O_2$ consumption in patients who remain agitated or who fight the ventilator

*Respiratory Secretions*

- Adequate IV hydration may aid in keeping secretions liquefied, easy to suction.
- Always humidify inspired gas to decrease viscosity of secretions and minimize trauma to mucous membranes.
- Use frequent tracheal suction, nasotracheal suction, or cough and deep breath exercises to eliminate secretions.
- Smokers always have heavy secretions. Treat with albuterol (5 mg/mL) mini-nebs 0.5 cc in 2.5 cc saline q4–6h.
- Mucolytic agents may be used in mini-nebulizer (mini-neb) form to treat tenacious secretions; e.g., Mucomyst (acetyl-eysteine 200 mg/mL) 1 mL mixed with 0.5 mL Albuterol (5 mg/mL) in 1.5 mL saline administered as a mini-neb q4–6h or PRN.

*Monitoring*

Patients on a ventilator ideally should have the following:
- $O_2$ sat monitor
- End tidal $CO_2$ monitor
- Arterial line (for frequent ABG testing)
- Pulmonary artery catheter in cases of high PEEP (≥10 cm $H_2O$), cardiac disease, or need to monitor fluid status

**Pulmonary Edema**

*Types*—Cardiogenic and noncardiogenic (ARDS).

*Cardiogenic Pulmonary Edema*—Due to pump failure, which causes increased intravascular pressures in the pulmonary vascular system. Fluid is "pushed" out into the pulmonary interstitium.

*ARDS*—Microvessels in the pulmonary system become "leaky" due to systemic inflammatory process. Fluid "leaks" out into the pulmonary interstitium.

- Swan-Ganz catheter is used to diagnose the type of pulmonary edema. If wedge pressure is <15, then is likely ARDS. If wedge pressure is >15, then is likely cardiogenic pulmonary edema.
- Treat cardiogenic pulmonary edema with diuretics and inotropes.
- Treat ARDS with ventilatory support, using PEEP, pressure support, and/or permissive hypercapnea (low TV with high rate).

---

**FACT BOX 20**

ARDS is defined by a $PaO_2$ to $FiO_2$ ratio <200.

---

# 10

# Cardiovascular System

**Parameters**

The cardiac system functions to pump blood (right ventricle) to the lungs for oxygenation and to distribute oxygenated blood (left ventricle) peripherally for normal cell respiration and function. The basic components of the cardiovascular system are:

*Preload*—Represents volume status and venous return

*Afterload*—Correlates with peripheral vascular resistance and blood pressure

*Contractility*—Correlates with stroke volume, cardiac output

*Hgb/Hct*—Adequate hemoglobin/hematocrit necessary in terms of $O_2$ carrying capacity

## *Optimization of Cardiovascular Parameters*

When physiologic control mechanisms of the body fail to function properly or have been altered by surgery or trauma, it is necessary to medically optimize cardiovascular parameters to re-establish adequate tissue perfusion and oxygenation.

- Volume load to support preload (to increase intravascular volume).
- Afterload adjustment: Increase with vasopressors, decrease with vasodilators as needed.
- Correct hypoxemia with supplemental $O_2$ or mechanical ventilation.
- Correct anemia with transfusion of PRBCs.
- Use inotropic drugs to increase "pump" action of heart (i.e., contractility).

48

## Monitoring

*Arterial Line*—For continuous blood pressure measurement and access for repeated arterial blood gases (ABGs)

*Pulmonary Artery Catheter (PAC)*—To monitor cardiac performance and cardiac filling (aka Swan-Ganz catheter)

### Data Obtained From Placement of a PAC

**TABLE 10.1**
**PAC Normal Values**

| Variable | Normal Value |
| --- | --- |
| Central venous pressure (CVP) | 5 mm Hg |
| Pulmonary capillary wedge pressure (PCWP) | 10–15 mm Hg |
| Cardiac output (CO) | 5 L/min |
| Cardiac index (CI) | 2.2–4.0 L/min/m$^2$ |
| Systemic vascular resistance (SVR) | 1000 dyne-sec/cm$^5$ |
| Mixed venous $O_2$ saturation ($SvO_2$) | 65–75% |

*Interpretation of PAC Data*

*Preload*—PCWP, CVP

*Afterload*—SVR

*Contractility*—CO, CI, ventricular function curve (graph of cardiac output versus PCWP)

*$O_2$ Utilization*—$SvO_2$

---

**FACT BOX 21**

Cardiac index (CI) is a normalized value and determined by the following:
CI = CO/BMI (BMI = body mass index)

---

*Differential Diagnosis of Low Cardiac Output*

- If low PCWP, high SVR, *think* hypovolemia. Treat with IV fluids.
- If high PCWP, normal SVR, *think* primary cardiac failure. Treat with inotropes (e.g., dobutamine).

- If high PCWP and SVR, *think* failure secondary to vasoconstriction. Treat with vasodilator (e.g., nitroprusside).

**Cardiac Medications in ICU**

Dobutamine 5–25 mcg/kg/min
- Increases contractility
- Decreases SVR (i.e., vasodilate)
- Decreases PCWP
- Frequently used to augment cardiac output or cardiac index

Amrinone (Inocor) 5–25 mcg/kg/min
- Increases contractility (i.e., CI)
- Decreases SVR (i.e., vasodilate)
- Decreases PCWP

Dopamine
- Renal vasodilator (doses <5 mcg/kg/min)
- Increases contractility (doses 5–10 mcg/kg/min
- Increases SVR (peripheral vasoconstrictor doses 10–20 mcg/kg/min)

Phenylephrine 40–60 mcg/min
- Increases afterload (vasoconstrictor)
- Increases blood pressure

Norepinephrine 2–4 mcg/min
- Vasoconstrictor
- Increases blood pressure
- Increases contractility

Nitroglycerin 5–20 mcg/min
- Arterial and venous vasodilator
- Decreases afterload (SVR)
- Decreases preload (CVP)

Nitroprusside 0.02–0.7 mg/min
- Arterial and venous vasodilator
- Decreases afterload (SVR)
- Decreases preload (CVP)

# 11

# Shock

*Definition of Shock*—Any situation in which $O_2$ delivery to the body as a whole is inadequate to meet metabolic demand.

## Types of Shock

*Hypovolemic*—Sudden volume loss
*Cardiogenic*—"Pump" failure
*Septic*—Massive vasodilation due to action of cytokines on vascular bed
*Neurogenic*—Massive vasodilation due to loss of sympathetic tone
*Anaphylactic*—Vascular leakiness, massive vasodilation, severe bronchospasm

## Management of Shock

- Treatment of shock must be rapid and aggressive. Morbidity and mortality increase linearly with delay in treatment.
- If the patient is assumed to be volume deficient for whatever reason, fluid resuscitation is indicated before pharmacologic treatment is initiated.

## Hypovolemic Shock

Hypervolemic shock results from sudden decrease of intravascular volume.

FACT BOX 22

Water moves into areas of high oncotic pressure, (e.g., burned tissue, retroperitoneum during pancreatitis).

### Etiology

- Hemorrhage
- Bowel obstruction (prolonged vomiting and third spacing)
- Burns
- Pancreatitis

### Signs

- Hypotension
- Tachycardia
- Vasoconstriction (skin cold to the touch)
- Diaphoresis (skin feels clammy)
- Mental status changes (confusion, combativeness)
- Decreased urine output
- Decreased CVP, PCWP, and CO

**TABLE 11.1**
**Signs of Acute Blood Loss**

| % Blood Volume Lost | Pulse | Systolic BP | Pulse Pressure (SBP-DBP) | Capillary Refill | Mental Status | Urine Output |
|---|---|---|---|---|---|---|
| <15 | Normal | Normal | Normal | Normal | Normal | Normal |
| 15–30 | >100 | Normal | Decrease | Delayed | Anxious | 20–30 mL/h |
| 30–40 | >120 | Decrease | Decrease | Delayed | Confused | 20 mL/h |
| >40 | >140 | Decrease | Decrease | Absent | Lethargic | Anuria |

### Management

- Aggressive IVF resuscitation, classically with LR (use NS if proven anuric, hyperkalemic, or if known renal failure).
- Transfusion of PRBC is indicated if ongoing hemorrhage or if >30% blood volume lost.

- Surgical therapy to stop hemorrhage, correct bowel obstruction, etc.
- Place Foley catheter; use urine output as a rough indicator of adequacy of resuscitation.
- PAC (Swan-Ganz) monitoring is necessary for elderly patients or for patients with decreased cardiac or renal function.

## Cardiogenic Shock

Cardiogenic shock is cardiac insufficiency ("pump" failure) resulting in inadequate "whole body" perfusion.

### Etiology

- MI
- Cardiac contusion
- Cardiac tamponade

### Symptoms and Signs

- Hypotension
- Distended neck veins
- Dyspnea (shortness of breath)
- Rales
- Loud pulmonic component of S2
- Cardiac gallop
- Pulsus alternans (fluctuating pulse pressure)
- Decreased CO and increased PCWP
- Peripheral vasoconstriction (skin cold to the touch)
- Cardiomegaly and pulmonary venous congestion seen on CXR

### Management

- Intubate—Use mechanical ventilation to put patient at complete rest, thus decreasing $O_2$ demand.
- PAC (Swan-Ganz) monitoring necessary in all cases.
- Inotropes—To increase "pump" performance. Goal is CI of >2.2 L/min $\times$ m$^2$.
- IVF—Conservative (slow) IVF resuscitation is indicated only if volume depleted.

- Diuresis—If increased PCWP, normal BP.
- Vasodilators—If normal PCWP, increased SVR.
- If all else fails, use of an intra-aortic balloon pump is indicated.

---

**FACT BOX 23**

Intra-aortic balloon pump has two actions:
- Decreases afterload as the balloon deflates during systole
- Increases coronary perfusion as the balloon inflates during diastole

---

**Septic Shock**

Septic shock is caused by decreased vascular resistance (massive vasodilation, decreased intravascular volume relative to the sudden increase in vascular capacity) secondary to bacterial toxins that activate the inflammatory cascade. The body's own inflammatory mediators (e.g., cytokines) cause massive vasodilation, microvascular pooling, and increased capillary permeability.

*Etiology*

- Gram-negative septicemia most common
- Gram-positive sepsis
- Reperfusion of ischemic limb or ischemic gut
- Pancreatitis

*Early Signs*

- Hypotension that responds to pressors
- Tachycardia
- Peripheral vasodilation (full bounding pulses, skin warm to the touch)
- Increased cardiac output (often 15 L/min)
- Decreased SVR, PCWP, CVP
- Normal to low urine output
- Fever

*Late Signs*

- Vasoconstriction
- Decreased cardiac output
- Greatly decreased urine output
- Hypotension unresponsive to pressors

*Laboratory Findings*

- Hypoglycemia
- Respiratory alkalosis
- Leukocytosis early leading to leukopenia later
- Thrombocytopenia

*Management*

- Massive IVF resuscitation (often 15 or more liters in the first 24 hours).
- Pan culture (blood, urine, sputum) and start empiric broad antibiotic treatment.
- Identify focus of infection and treat.
- Urgent surgical drainage of intra-abdominal abscess (diagnosed usually with CT scan).
- Surgical excision of all dead tissue (e.g., limbs, intestine).
- Place Foley catheter; use urine output as a rough indicator of adequacy of resuscitation.
- PAC (Swan-Ganz) monitoring necessary for all patients, especially for elderly patients or for patients with decreased cardiac or renal function.

### Neurogenic Shock

Neurogenic shock is inadequate tissue perfusion due to a loss of sympathetic vasoconstrictive tone (massive vasodilation).

*Etiology*

- Spinal trauma
- Spinal anesthesia

### Signs

- Hypotension
- Bradycardia
- Vasodilation (skin warm to the touch)
- Decreased SVR, CO, PCWP, CVP
- Loss of sensory and motor function below the lesion (e.g., paraplegia)

### Management

- IVF resuscitation classically with LR
- Pressors to provide chemical vasoconstriction peripherally
- Place Foley catheter; use urine output as a rough indicator of adequacy of resuscitation
- PAC monitoring necessary for elderly patients or for patients with decreased cardiac or renal function

## Anaphylactic Shock

Anaphylactic shock is inadequate tissue perfusion due to massive vasodilation and increased vascular permeability as a result of allergen exposure.

### Etiology

- Medications
- Bee sting (Hymenoptera venom)
- Wasp sting
- Food allergies (e.g., nuts, seafood)
- Blood transfusions
- Latex allergies (usually becomes apparent in the operating room)

### Signs and Symptoms

- Laryngeal edema (stridor)
- Respiratory smooth muscle contraction (bronchial spasm)
- Hypotension
- Tachycardia
- Hypoxemia

- Urticaria (purple splotches)
- Angioedema
- Nausea, vomiting, diarrhea

### *Management*

- Establish patent airway.
- IVF resuscitation.
- Epinephrine.
- Benadryl.
- Steroids if needed.
- Remove the offending allergen.

# 12

# Advanced Cardiac Life Support (ACLS)

**Ventricular Fibrillation (VF)/
Pulseless Ventricular Tachycardia (VT)**

*Ventricular Fibrillation/Tachycardia*

ABCs (airway, breathing, circulation)
CPR until defibrillator/monitor attached
Defibrillate (up to 3 times)
- 200 J
- 300 J
- 360 J
Resume CPR if VF/VT persists.
Intubate as soon as possible.
Obtain IV access.
Begin pushing drugs.

*Medications*

*Epinephrine*—1 mg IV push q3–5m
  May be given endotracheally if dissolved in 9 cc NS
*Amiodarone*—300 mg IV, may give 2nd dose of 150 mg IV
  (max 2.2g/24 hours)
*Lidocaine*—1–1.5 mg/kg IV push q3–5m
  3 mg/kg maximum dose

*Bretylium*—5 mg/kg IV push. Repeat in 5 minutes at 10 mg/kg.
   30 mg/kg maximum dose
*Procainamide*—30 mg/min IV drip
   17 mg/kg maximum dose (approximately 40 minutes at
   30 mg/min)

NOTE: Use CPR to circulate drugs for 45 seconds after each dose, then defibrillate at 360 J and recheck pulse after each defibrillation.


**Pulseless Electrical Activity (PEA)**

Begin/continue CPR.
Intubate as soon as possible.
Obtain IV access.
NO defibrillation!
Assess blood flow with Doppler if possible.


*Consider Possible Etiologies (and Treat If Applicable)*

Hypoxia (ventilate with 100% $O_2$)
Hypovolemia (rapid fluid infusion)
Cardiac tamponade (pericardiocentesis)
Tension pneumothorax (needle decompression using a 14-gauge
   catheter in the 2nd costal interspace in the mid-clavicular line)
Hypothermia (warm the patient)
Pulmonary embolism (surgery to remove thrombus)
Drug overdose, e.g., tricyclics, digitalis, β-blockers, calcium chan-
   nel blockers
Hyperkalemia (calcium IV, bicarbonate IV, 10 units insulin with
   1 amp D50 IV, furosemide [Lasix])
Acidosis (bicarbonate IV, fluid bolus)
Myocardial infarction (MI)


*Medications*

*Epinephrine*—1 mg IV push q3–5m
*Atropine*—(if absolute bradycardia <60 bpm) 1 mg IV q3–5min
   (0.04 mg/kg) (maximum dose approximately 3 mg total)

**Asystole**

Begin CPR.
Intubate as soon as possible.
Obtain IV access.
Confirm asystole on two or more leads.
Immediate transcutaneous pacing.

### Consider Possible Etiologies (and Treat If Applicable)

Hypoxia (ventilate with 100% $O_2$)
Hyperkalemia (calcium IV, bicarbonate IV, 10 units insulin with
   one amp D50W IV, furosemide [Lasix])
Hypokalemia (K+ runs)
Acidosis (bicarbonate IV, fluid bolus)
Overdose
Hypothermia (warm the patient)

### Medications

*Epinephrine*—1 mg IV push q3–5min
*Atropine*—1 mg IV q3–5min (maximum dose approximately
   3 mg)

**Bradycardia (Pulse <60 beats per minute [bpm])**

ABCs, secure the airway.
Start $O_2$.
Obtain IV access.
Monitor patient's ECG, pulse oximeter, blood pressure.
Measure vital signs.
Perform directed H&P.
Obtain 12-lead ECG and CXR.

### If Patient Is Symptomatic

Atropine—1 mg IV push (approximately 3 mg maximum dose)
Transcutaneous pacing (TCP) for patients with type II second
   degree or third degree heart block
Dopamine drip 5–20 mcg/kg/min
Epinephrine drip 2–10 mcg/min

**Tachycardia**

*Tachycardia*

ABCs.
Start $O_2$.
Obtain IV access.
Monitor patient's ECG, pulse oximeter, blood pressure.
Measure vital signs.
Perform directed H&P.
Obtain 12-lead ECG and CXR.

*Atrial Fibrillation/Atrial Flutter*

Diltiazem 0.25 mg/kg.
Verapamil 5 mg IV push.
Beta blockers.
Load with digoxin.
Procainamide, quinidine, start heparin.

*Paroxysmal Supraventricular Tachycardia (PSVT)*

Vagal maneuvers
Adenosine 6 mg rapid IV push
Adenosine 12 mg rapid push, may repeat once after 1–2 minutes
Adenosine 12 mg push verapamil 2.5–5 mg IV, may repeat after
    15 minutes

*Wide Complex Tachycardia*

Lidocaine 1–1.5 mg/kg IV push
Lidocaine 0.5–0.75 mg/kg IV (maximum 3 mg/kg)
Adenosine 6 mg IV push
Adenosine 12 mg IV push, may repeat once in 1–2 minutes
Procainamide 20–30 mg/minute
Bretylium 5–10 mg/kg over 10 minutes (maximum 30 mg/kg
    over 24 hours)

### *Ventricular Tachycardia*

Lidocaine 1–1.5 mg/kg IV push
Lidocaine 0.5–0.75 mg/kg IV push (maximum 3 mg/kg dose)
Procainamide 20–30 mg/min (maximum 40 minutes)
Bretylium 5–10 mg/kg over 10 minutes (maximum 30 mg/kg)

# 13

# Preoperative Assessment and Workup

**American Society of Anesthesiology (ASA) Scale**

Measure of physiologic well-being. Mortality increases with increased ASA score.

*ASA I*—Healthy patient (predict 0% mortality)

*ASA II*—One systemic disease well controlled; does not affect daily activity (predict minimum mortality)

*ASA III*—Multisystem disease, well controlled but limits activity

*ASA IV*—Severe incapacitating disease with poor control, constant threat to life (greatly increased mortality predicted)

*ASA V*—Moribund patient not expected to survive 24 hours with or without surgery

*ASA VI*—Brain-dead organ donor

*Subclass E*—Indicates emergent procedure. Emergent surgeries can have double the mortality of elective procedures.

**Risk Factors for Increased Perioperative Morbidity/Mortality**

*Age*

- Increasing age produces changes in physiologic responses to surgery and stress.

### Cardiovascular

- Coronary artery disease (CAD), worse if there are symptoms of angina
- Congestive heart failure (CHF)
- Arrhythmias
- Peripheral vascular disease (PVD)
- HTN
- Recent MI presents an increased risk of perioperative infarct or sudden death

**TABLE 13.1**
**Cardiac Risk Following MI**

| Time Since MI | Risk |
| --- | --- |
| 0–3 months | 6% |
| 4–6 months | 2% |
| >6 months | 1% |

FACT BOX 24

Patients should wait at least 3–6 months after an MI before having elective surgery if possible.

### Respiratory

- Smoking, especially >20-pack a year history (any history of smoking, e.g., marijuana, cigars, increases risk)
- Obesity
- COPD ($pO_2$ <60, $pCO_2$ >50, $FEV_1/FVC$ <70%)
- Pulmonary hypertension
- Respiratory risk factors have the greatest impact after thoracic surgery, moderate impact after upper abdominal surgery, and least impact after lower abdominal surgery

### Renal

- BUN >50, Cr >3.0
- History of renal insufficiency

## Hepatic

- Cirrhosis, especially Child's class B or C
- Active hepatitis

## Endocrine

- Diabetes
- Steroid use
- Thyroid disease

## Preoperative Workup for Elective Surgery

Begins with history, physical exam, and assessment of the patient

### Preoperative Labs and Tests

- CBC, UA, Chem-7, PT/PTT
- CXR and ECG if >40 years old or if indicated otherwise
- Blood type and cross for appropriate number of units for surgery being performed

### Cardiovascular Disease

- Evaluate patients with known CAD with ECG, stress thallium, or ECHO preoperatively. If patient unable to exercise, substitute dobutamine thallium for stress thallium.
- Treat with perioperative nitroglycerin if workup shows cardiac ischemia and if coronary artery bypass is not feasible.

### Hypertension

- No increased risk with stable or mild hypertension with diastolic <110 mm Hg.
- Continue antihypertensive medication with sips of $H_2O$ (even while NPO prior to procedure).
- Discontinue any monoamine oxidase (MAO) inhibitors 2 weeks prior to surgery.
- New onset hypertension or malignant hypertension requires further workup prior to surgery to locate cause and to evaluate for possible end organ damage (renal, cardiovascular, retinal, cerebral).

### *Pulmonary Disease*

- Need to quit smoking for at least 8 weeks prior to surgery to decrease the risk of pulmonary complications.
- ABG on room air if indicated by severity of pulmonary dysfunction (e.g., >20-pack a year smoking history, dyspnea on exertion or with climbing 1–2 flights of stairs, or abnormal physical exam).
- Preop room air ABG and/or pulmonary function tests (PFTs) necessary for all elective thoracic and cardiac surgery.
- Increase bronchodilator use preoperatively. If not using bronchodilators at home, start albuterol inhaler, 2–4 puffs qid.
- Chest physiotherapy, coughing, deep breathing, and incentive spirometry for several days preop may improve the patient's respiratory toilet and vital capacity.
- Patients with documented bronchitis or pneumonia should have all elective procedures postponed and pulmonary infections treated.

### *Renal Disease*

- Correct any underlying problems, including:
  - Abnormal electrolytes
  - Depleted volume status.
- Schedule hemodialysis for the evening prior to or morning of surgery.

#### *Preoperative Antibiotics*

- Given 30 minutes prior to incision. Examples include:
  - Cefazolin (Ancef, Kefzol) 1 g IV
  - Vancomycin 1 g IV in PCN allergic patients

#### *Preoperative Antibiotics Indicated For:*

- Clean contaminated (GI, GU, respiratory, GYN) procedures
- Contaminated cases (perforated appendicitis, perforated colon, trauma)
- Placement of any prosthetic material
- Patients with preexisting synthetic grafts or materials
- Patients with preexisting valvular heart disease

### Other Preoperative Orders

*Nutrition*—NPO after midnight except for meds with sips $H_2O$ (need 6–8 hours to empty stomach to decrease risk of aspiration).

*Fluids*—Preop maintenance fluids: D5 2 NS with 20 mEq KCl/L at calculated rate (4/2/1 rule).

*Medications*—Continue maintenance medications with sips $H_2O$. Add an $H_2$ blocker and sleeping medication for patient comfort.

*IV Lines*—Need at least one 18 G IV line for anesthetic drugs and fluids. Arterial lines and central venous lines are indicated for larger operations or sicker patients.

*Enterostomal Therapist*—Mark possible stoma sites.

*Steroids*
- Indications for perioperative steroids
  ○ Patient currently taking steroids or has taken steroids within the past year
  ○ Adrenal insufficiency
  ○ Previous surgery of the adrenal or pituitary glands
  ○ History of renal cell carcinoma resection.
- Normal cortisol output is 10–30 mg/day.
- Patients require 100 mg of corticosteroid per day after stresses such as surgery.
- Dosage: 100 mg hydrocortisone IV OCTOR, 100 mg IV in RR, then 100 mg IV q6 for 24 hours. Decrease to 50 mg IV q6 for 24 hours and then taper.

### Bowel Prep

All abdominal surgery should be preceded by a complete bowel prep. Both mechanical cleansing of the bowel contents and antibiotics to decrease bacterial counts are necessary.

### Options

*Mechanical Preps*

(Clear liquid diet the day before surgery and NPO p MN. Mechanical preps should be done prior to antibiotic administration.)

1. GoLYTELY (polyethylene glycol solution) 4 liters over 4 hours the day before surgery.
2. Bisacodyl 10 mg tab 4 PO. Then after 4 hours Fleet Phospho-soda 30 mL followed by 8 oz water. Then repeat q4h × 1.
3. Magnesium citrate 1 bottle q4h × 2.

*Antibiotic Prep*

• Neomycin 1 g and erythromycin base 1 g—1 pm, 2 pm, and 11 pm prior to surgery

# 14

# Surgical Complications

**Pulmonary System**

*Atelectasis*

Collapse of alveoli due to inadequate lung expansion. This can be the result of poor ventilation during surgery or difficulty with deep inspiration and cough secondary to pain after surgery.

*Symptoms and Signs*

- Fever
- Decreased breath sounds
- Tachypnea
- Tachycardia

---

FACT BOX **25**

Atelectasis is the most common cause of postoperative fever in the first 48 hours.

---

*Management*

- Up out of bed (OOB) to chair, ambulate
- Cough and deep breath
- Incentive spirometer
- Chest percussion and postural drainage

### *Respiratory Failure*

Inadequate tissue oxygenation secondary to decreased pulmonary gas exchange. Two main causes: problems with oxygenation of blood (atelectasis, pneumonia, pulmonary edema, pulmonary embolus, or hypovolemia) or problems with mechanical work of breathing (narcotic overdose, impaired respiratory drive, increased intra-abdominal pressure, pneumothorax, or hemothorax).

*Symptoms and Signs:*

- Respiratory rate >25 or <10
- $pO_2$ <60, cyanosis, confusion, agitation
- $pCO_2$ >50

*Management*

- Treatment of true respiratory failure requires endotracheal intubation and mechanical ventilation

### *Pulmonary Embolus*

Results from a blood clot lodging in a pulmonary artery. Clot usually arises due to deep venous thrombosis (DVT) of the calf, thigh, or iliac/pelvic vessels. Factors that increase risk are:

- Immobility (stasis)
- Obesity
- Oral contraceptives (hypercoagulable state)
- Smoking (endothelial injury)
- Malignancy (hypercoagulable state)
- Polycythemia
- Pelvic surgery (stasis, local compression)
- Pelvic fracture (endothelial injury)
- History of previous DVT

---

**FACT BOX 26**

Virchow's Triad
- Stasis
- Endothelial injury
- Hypercoagulable state

---

*Symptoms and Signs*

- Sudden onset of dyspnea, tachypnea, hypotension, chest pain, fever, or loud $S_2$.
- Supraventricular tachycardia.
- Lower extremities may be tender or edematous (due to DVT).
- ABG identifies decreased $pO_2$ and $pCO_2$.

*Diagnosis*

- Definitive diagnosis is made by pulmonary arteriography (arteriography also allows for intra-arterial infusion of thrombolytic agents).
- Ventilation perfusion (V/Q) scan, which shows high probability, is also acceptable to make the diagnosis.

*Management*

- Heparin anticoagulation, convert to warfarin (Coumadin) when stable
- Cardiac support with inotropes and oxygen in the ICU
- Thrombolytic therapy
- Inferior vena cava filter for patients who are not candidates for anticoagulation or who sustain a pulmonary embolus while anticoagulated
- Thoracotomy, embolectomy (high mortality)

**Renal System**

*Acute Renal Failure (ARF)*

Potentially reversible deterioration in renal function that is sudden in onset and is sufficient to cause nitrogenous waste accumulation in body fluids

*Etiology*

- Prerenal—Most common cause in surgical patients is intravascular volume depletion. Others include CHF, shock, cardiac tamponade, and renal artery stenosis.

- Postrenal—Urinary obstruction usually due to benign prostatic hypertrophy or clogged Foley catheter
- Renal—Acute tubular necrosis with nearly 60% of all perioperative cases related to a nephrotoxin

*Nephrotoxins*

If your patient develops signs and symptoms of renal failure, make sure to D/C all nephrotoxic medications and limit IV contrast.

- Aminoglycosides, amphotericin B
- Nonsteroidal anti-inflammatory drugs (NSAIDs)
- ACE inhibitors
- Radiocontrast
- Intravascular cellular debris, e.g., myoglobin
- Some $H_2$ blockers (Pepcid)

---

**FACT BOX 27**

Oliguria is <0.5 mL/kg/h or less than the amount needed to excrete daily osmolar load.

---

*Urine Output*

- Anuria <100 cc/day
- Oliguria <500 cc/day

*Labs*

- BMP, urinalysis (UA)—Look for eosinophils in the urine.
- Spot urine for Na, Cr, and osmolarity. 24-hour urine will be more accurate.

Fractional excretion of sodium (FeNa) helps to differentiate cause of a ARF as pre- or postrenal.

- FeNa <1% suggests prerenal cause.
- FeNa >2% suggests renal or postrenal cause.

---

FACT BOX **28**

Indications for dialysis
- Acidosis
- Hyperkalemia
- Uremic pericarditis
- Fluid overload
- Encephalopathy

---

*Management*

- Remove all $K^+$ from IVF.
- Change Foley catheter.
- Fluid challenge with 500 cc bolus of NS.
- Stop all nephrotoxic drugs.
- Address underlying problems and treat if possible.

Recovery time for ARF is a few days to 1 month with up to 10% mortality rate. 10% of patients will have continued renal dysfunction.

**GI System**

*Adynamic Ileus*

Loss of normal peristalsis, most common after abdominal surgery, can last from 24 hours to 7 days or longer postop. Postop return of normal bowel motility usually follows a predictable course:
- Small bowel motility, 24 hours
- Gastric motility, 48 hours
- Colonic motility, 3–7 days

---

FACT BOX **29**

Most of intestinal gas (>80%) is secondary to swallowed air. Flatus generally indicates transit of air from the mouth to the anus and suggests return of bowel function.

---

*Symptoms*

- Nausea
- Vomiting, bilious emesis
- Abdominal distention

*Management*

- Patient should be kept NPO until bowel function returns.
- IVF.
- NGT decompression if nausea and vomiting persist.
- For procedures not involving the GI system, some surgeons recommend stimulating the bowel with liquid diet within 24 hours regardless of degree of bowel function.
- TPN if prolonged (lasting more than 5 days).

## Surgical Infection

A surgical infection is either the result of surgery or an infection that requires surgical intervention. For a true infection to occur, a series of events must take place.

- An inoculum of pathogens of sufficient number and virulence to produce infection must be delivered to the site of infection. In general, >1000 colony-forming units is adequate to colonize a wound, but $10^5$ bacteria/mm$^3$ on tissue culture suggests an established infection.
- A sufficient medium must be available for pathogens to thrive in. These include blood, necrotic tissue, seroma, or healthy tissue with diminished resistance.
- Any alteration in normal host resistance whether local or systemic predisposes to infection.

### Symptoms and Signs

Assess patients for signs and symptoms of infection daily using history and physical exam.

*General local response to infection*

- Pain (dolor)
- Erythema (rubor)

- Warmth (calor)
- Swelling (tumor)
- Loss of function

*Systemic Response*

- Fever
- Chills
- Tachycardia
- Tachypnea
- Leukocytosis or leukopenia

## Management

*The three Ds*

- Debridement (remove dead tissue)
- Drainage (remove pus)
- Diversion (divert stool flow if needed to keep the wound clean)

### Common Bacteria and Antibiotic Selection

As a commentary to the following section, it is important to note that antibiotic selection cannot be made from a book. The best management of any infectious agent is to identify the organism and determine sensitivities to therapy. Then the antibiotic with the narrowest spectrum is employed to treat the infection.

### Surgical Infection and Antibiotic Therapy

1. Collect *appropriate* cultures (sputum, bronchial alveolar lavage (BAL), urine, blood, wound)
2. Initiate *brief broad spectrum* therapy if necessary (i.e., septic, hypoxic, hypotensive, etc.) for 24–48 hours
3. *Narrow spectrum* of antibiotic by bacterial identification and *sensitivities*

### Gram-Positive Cocci

Staphylococcus aureus

- Location: Wounds, incisions, central line, carbuncles, breast abscess
- Rx: Penicillin, cephalosporin, macrolide, tetracycline, Vancomycin

---

**FACT BOX 30**

- *Staphylococcus aureus* is the most common cause of nosocomial bacteremia.
- *Staphylococcus aureus* is the most common bacteria associated with wound infections.

---

Staphylococcus epidermidis

- Location: Central line infection, vascular graft infection.
- Rx: Remove line. If needed, treat with cephalosporin or vancomycin.
- Long-term antibiotic suppression with cephalexin (Keflex) may suffice to treat *S. epidermidis* vascular graft infection. For severe infections, removal of the graft is necessary.

Streptococcus pyogenes

- Location: Cellulites, folliculitis, glomuleronephritis
- Rx: Penicillin G, V, erythromycin

Streptococcus faecalis *(Enterococcus)*

- Location: Intra-abdominal infections, biliary tract infections, UTI
- Rx: Penicillin + aminoglycoside (e.g., ampicillin and gentamycin), Unasyn, Zosyn
- Vancomycin-resistant Enterococcus is associated with *S. faecalis* and *S. faecium*

Streptococcus pneumoniae

- Location: Pneumonia, sepsis, meningitis
- Rx: Penicillin G, erythromycin, ciprofloxacin

Streptococcus viridens

- Location: Subacute endocarditis
- Rx: Penicillin, Augmentin, Cipro

### Gram-Positive Rods (Bacilli)

Clostridium perfringens

- Location: Gas gangrene, myonecrosis
- Rx: Debridement, penicillin

Clostridium difficile

- Location: Pseudomembranous colitis
- Rx: Metronidazole, oral vancomycin

---

**FACT BOX 31**

Any patient requiring an increase in narcotics for incisional pain should be suspected of having clostridial infection.

---

### Gram-Negative Cocci

Haemophilus influenzae

- Location: Pneumonia
- Rx: Kefzol

### Gram-Negative Rods (Bacilli)

Escherichia coli, Proteus *species,* Klebsiella pneumoniae, Serratia, Enterobacter

- Location: Intra-abdominal infections, nosocomial pneumonia, abscess, UTI

- Rx: First-, second-, third-generation cephalosporin, penicillin, ampicillin, sulfonamides

### *Obligate Aerobic Gram-Negative Rods*

Pseudomonas aeruginosa

- Location: Nosocomial pneumonia, bacteremia, ventilator dependent. Common gram-negative nosocomial infection.
- Rx: Piperacillin, ticarcillin, ciprofloxacin

Acinetobacter

- Location: Nosocomial pneumonia, intra-abdominal infections, soft tissue infections
- Rx: Aztreonam, levofloxacin, piperacillin/tazobactam, ceftazidime, imipenem, ciprofloxacin, dual therapy often required

---

**FACT BOX 32**

- The most common inhabitants of the GI tract are anaerobes.
- The most important factor in lowering bacterial counts in the gut is mechanical removal with preoperative bowel prep.

---

*Anaerobes*

*Bacteroides fragilis, Clostridium perfringens*
*Clostridium tetani*
*Clostridium difficile*

- Location: Intra-abdominal infections, abscess, gas gangrene, pseudomembranous colitis
- Rx: Metronidazole, vancomycin (PO)

**FACT BOX 33**

*C. difficile* colitis is a common cause of diarrhea in patients who have received antibiotic therapy. Always check for *C. diff* toxin in the stool before initiating antidiarrheals. Failure to do so could lead to toxic megacolon and perforation.

### Pneumonia

#### Community Acquired

- *Streptococcus pneumoniae*
- *Mycoplasma pneumoniae*
- *H. influenzae*
- Legionella
- Chlamydia

#### Nosocomial

- Enteric gram-negative rods
- *Pseudomonas*
- *Staphylococcus*

#### Common GI Infections

- *Escherichia coli*
- *Salmonella typhi*
- *Salmonella enteritidis*
- *Shigella* species
- *Campylobacter jejuni*

### Classification of Surgical Infections

#### Cellulitis

Local inflammatory process without extensive tissue necrosis or purulent exudate

*Etiology*

- Most common cause is *Streptococcus* or *Staphylococcus*. The more virulent form of a *Streptococcus* infection is called erysipelas.

*Treatment*

- Elevation, warm compresses, and IV antibiotics (e.g., ampicillin, Unasyn, Kefzol)

### Phlegmon

Diffuse inflammation with scattered foci of necrotic tissue and accumulated pus. Initially presents as a cellulitis but progresses to more extensive tissue destruction.

*Etiology*

- Most common cause is *Streptococcus* or *Staphylococcus.*

*Treatment*

- Elevation, rest, and appropriate IV antibiotics. If extensive tissue necrosis is present, then surgical debridement will be required.

### Abscess

An inflammatory process consisting of a pus-filled cavity surrounded by a wall of granulation tissue

*Etiology*

- *Staphylococcus* and various other aerobic gram-negative rods and anaerobes

*Treatment*

- Antibiotics only play a secondary role in the treatment of bacteremia or septicemia that may result from advanced progression of the abscess or during manipulation of the abscess during drainage. The basic treatment for any abscess is surgical drainage.

### Gangrene

Infectious gangrene is caused by the action of microbial enzymes directly on healthy tissue or indirectly by the thrombosis of nutrient blood vessels.

*Aerobic Gangrene*—Usually caused by a virulent strain of hemolytic *Streptococcus*. Treatment requires wide debridement of all necrotic tissues and IV antibiotics (e.g., PCN).

*Anaerobic Gangrene*—Most commonly caused by the gas-forming bacillus *Clostridium perfringens*. Tissues become dark, cool, and areas of hemorrhage develop at the wound margins with intense pain and brackish watery discharge. Treatment requires wide surgical debridement and massive parenteral penicillin and anaerobic coverage (metronidazole).

*Necrotizing Fasciitis and Necrotizing Cellulitis*—Caused by synergistic activity of both anaerobes and aerobic gram-negative rods and are managed the same as anaerobic gangrene.

### Toxemia

The presence of toxins (endotoxins and exotoxins) in systemic circulation with disruptive influence on metabolic and/or physiologic host functions

#### Etiology

• Includes tetanus, diphtheria, pseudomonas

#### Treatment

• Remove source of toxin, massive doses of appropriate antibiotics (e.g., PCN) and antitoxins (e.g., tetanus toxoid) if available. Supportive fluid and electrolyte management may be necessary.

### Septicemia

The progression of bacteremia with propagation of blood-borne bacteria. Septicemia causes significant and profound systemic effects including peripheral pooling of blood, heart failure, coagulopathy.

*Treatment*

- Involves elimination of the bacterial focus of infection, antibiotics, and supportive measures (IVF, pressors, PAC monitoring)

## Spontaneous Bacterial Peritonitis

*Etiology*

- Most often is idiopathic, but may follow paracentesis or peritoneal lavage.
- Usually associated with cirrhosis, systemic lupus erythematosus (SLE), and ascites.
- Most common organism is *E. coli.*

*Treatment*

- Broad-spectrum antibiotics

## Intra-abdominal Abscess

Classic locations are subphrenic, subhepatic, lateral gutters, pelvic, and paracolic.

*Symptoms*

- Abdominal pain
- Spiking fevers

*Diagnosis*

- CT scan of abdomen and pelvis

*Treatment*

- Drainage and parenteral antibiotics. Drainage may be percutaneous or surgical (open).
- Subphrenic abscesses can be drained through a posterior 12th rib approach.

## Skin Infections

*Furuncle*—Begins as an infection of skin appendages (hair follicle, sebaceous gland) and progresses to an intradermal abscess with subcutaneous extension. *Staphylococcus* or *Streptococcus* are the usual pathogens. The furuncle usually will drain spontaneously after necrosing the overlying skin.

*Hidradenitis*—An infection of apocrine sweat glands in the axilla or groin area.

*Sebaceous Cysts*—Develop over the face, scalp, neck, and upper trunk and arise from obstruction of the sebaceous gland. Once acute infection resolves residual cyst and scar may be excised with an ellipse of overlying skin.

*Carbuncle*—More extensive infection of the dermis and subcutaneous tissue. Occurs most frequently in diabetics.

*Folliculitis*—*Staphylococcus* infection of the hair follicles in areas of dense thick hair growth (suprapubic, beard). Infection tends to persist until both local and systemic antibiotics are applied.

### Wound Infection

Increasing incisional pain with erythema, cellulitis, or presence of purulent discharge from the wound noted on physical exam. Superficial infections make up 75% of all wound infections.

- Onset 3–7 days postop
- *Staphylococcus* and *Streptococcus* most common organisms

---

**FACT BOX 34**

Wound infection within the first 24 hours is usually due to *Streptococcus* or *Clostridium*.

---

*Wound Infection Rates by Case Type*

- Clean <2%
- Clean-contaminated 7%
- Contaminated 15%
- Dirty/Infected 40%

*Management*

Remove sutures or staples from skin and subcutaneous tissue, open and drain the wound, and obtain cultures and sensitivities.

TABLE 14.1
**Characteristics of Wound Infections**

| Postop Day | Pathogen | Appearance | Signs/Symptoms |
|---|---|---|---|
| 1–3 | *Clostridium perfringens* | Brawny, cool, hemorrhagic | Sustained fever, leukocytosis, jaundice, intense incisional pain, crepitance |
| 1–3 | *Streptococcus* | Erythema, serous exudate | High spiking fever, leukocytosis, incision is warm and tender |
| 3–4 | *Staphylococcus* | Erythema, purulent exudate | High spiking fever, leukocytosis, incision is warm and tender |

Examine the underlying fascia for integrity. Pack wound with wet to dry saline dressings tid. May close wound secondarily when infection clears and granulation tissue is present.

### Wound Dehiscence

Divided into two categories: superficial and fascial.
*Superficial dehiscence*—Refers to nonhealing of skin and subcutaneous tissue. Treat with wet-to-dry dressing changes tid.
*Fascial dehiscence*—Has a 15% mortality and is the result of
  • Ischemia
  • Increased intra-abdominal pressure
  • Infection
  • Excessive tension
  • Technical error.

Treat with wound exploration, debridement, and tensionless closure under general anesthesia.

### Fever

Postoperative fever can be the result of many etiologies. Identification of the correct etiology is necessary for appropriate management. The most common causes of postoperative fever are the 6 Ws:
*Wind*—(Pulmonary) atelectasis, pneumonia
*Water*—UTI

*Wound*—Wound infection, cellulitis
*Walk*—DVT
*Wing (Waterway)*—Arms (catheters)—IV lines, PICC lines, central venous catheters
*Wonder Drugs*—Drug fever (PCN, ampicillin, etc.)

### Causes of Postop Fever

*0–48 Hours*

- Atelectasis
- Soft tissue infection with *Clostridium* or *Streptococcus*
- Leaky bowel anastomosis
- Aspiration pneumonia

*Day 3–6*

- UTI (discontinue Foley if possible)
- Wound infection
- IV site phlebitis (peripheral IVs should be changed every 2–3 days)
- Central venous catheter–related sepsis (remove catheter; if fever resolves, no antibiotics needed)

*Day 6–10*

- Intra-abdominal abscess (presents with spiking fevers)
- Deep venous thrombosis (7–10 days)
- Acalculous cholecystitis (especially in patients who are NPO)
- Sinusitis in patients with prolonged NG, or endotracheal intubation
- Perirectal abscess
- Drug fever

# 15

# On-Call Issues

On call, you will encounter many patient-care issues. Remember: Common things occur commonly. Basic rules are:

- Go to the bedside when the nurses call and examine the patient to rule out serious or life-threatening issues. Never trust assessments by others relayed over the phone.
- Avoid only treating symptoms while ignoring the underlying problem.
- Always call for help (upper-level resident or attending) if uncertain.

## Fever

### Etiology

Think about the 6 Ws:

*Wind:* Atelectasis

- Pulmonary atelectasis causes fever in the early postoperative period (0–48 hours postop). Treat with coughing, deep breathing, and incentive spirometry (C/DB/IS). Get the patient up out of bed to a chair.

*Water:* UTI (check UA)

*Wound:* Infection (look for erythema or crepitance)

*Walk:* DVT (check for calf tenderness)

*Wing/Waterway:* Peripheral and central venous catheters (look for erythema or purulence)

*Wonder Drugs:* Drug-induced fever

*Spiking Fevers:* Think abscess or endocarditis.
- Avoid treating fevers with acetaminophen (Tylenol) unless workup is in progress or a source is known.

### Workup for Fever of Unknown Origin

- Physical exam
- CBC with differential
- CXR
- UA with microscopic analysis
- Blood cultures × 2, 30 minutes apart
- Sputum culture
- Urine culture
- If previous abdominal surgery, CT scan of the abdomen and pelvis
- If severe headache, CT scan of the head and lumbar puncture
- If central line present, start new line or change over a wire and send tip for culture

### Nausea and Vomiting

In general, surgical patients with nausea and vomiting require GI decompression with a nasogastric tube. Do not blindly treat nausea and vomiting pharmacologically (e.g., with promethazine [Phenergan], odansetron [Zofran], prochlorperazine [Compazine]). Differential diagnosis includes ileus versus obstructive pathology.

### Management

- Make the patient NPO.
- Place NG tube, irrigate q2h with 30 mL NS, keep tube patent and sumping.
- Obtain acute abdominal series (flat and upright abdominal x-rays).
- Consider upper GI with small bowel follow-through using Gastrografin. Postanesthesia nausea can be treated with:
  - Odansetron [Zofran] (4 mg IV q6h prn), or
  - Promethazine [Phenergan] (12.5–25 mg IV q4–6h prn).

FACT BOX **35**

> Gastrografin is associated with significant pulmonary complications if aspirated and barium is associated with significant abdominal complications if expressed through a perforation.

## Low Urine Output

The most significant and valuable tool to assess volume status is the urine output (UOP). For most surgical patients a UOP >30cc/h indicates adequate intravascular volume (or preload).

### *Etiology*

*Hypovolemia (prerenal)*—Most common postoperative cause of decreased UOP, especially after large abdominal procedures. Treatment:
- Place Foley catheter.
- Bolus 1 L NS or LR IV. Can repeat bolus unless signs of overload present (crackles, hypoxia).
- If UOP improves with bolus, change IVF to LR at 2–3 times maintenance rate.
- If UOP does not improve, consider monitoring with Swan-Ganz catheter.

*Renal Failure*—Acute renal failure or acute tubular acidosis.
- CHEM-7 and assess BUN/Cr ratio
- Urine sodium to calculate FeNa (fractional excretion of sodium)
- May require emergent hemodialysis

*Obstruction (postrenal)*—Patients may have urinary retention, especially after spinal anesthesia or inguinal hernia repair. Indwelling Foley catheters can become obstructed.
- Place Foley catheter or change existing Foley catheter.
- If unable to change Foley catheter, irrigate existing Foley with 30 cc NS.

---

> | FACT BOX 36 |
>
> Urine output is usually increased on the third to fourth postoperative day secondary to mobilization of third space fluid.

## Pain Control

Patients do have significant incisional pain following surgery depending on the type and extent of the procedure. Look for signs of poorly controlled pain such as tachycardia and hypertension. Goal is to provide adequate pain control to maintain patient comfort without overmedicating. Narcotics do cause nausea with bolus dosing. Give bolus narcotics with small doses of promethazine (Phenergan) IV.

### Morphine Sulfate (MS)

- Patient-controlled anesthesia (PCA): (1 mg/1 mL), 1 mL IV q8min with 8 mg lockout over 1 hour
- 2–6 mg IV q1 2h
- 6–10 mg intramuscularly (IM) q2–4h
- Better long-term pain control with IM dosing (Note: IM route contraindicated in immunocompromised patients, diabetics, coagulopathic, etc.)
- Can add MS 1–3 mg IV q2h for breakthrough pain to other established regimen, e.g., patient on oral pain medications

### Meperidine (Demerol)

- PCA: (10 mg/1 mL), 1 mL IV q8min with 80-mg lockout over 1 hour
- 25–50 mg IV q3h
- 50–100 mg IM q4h (better long-term pain control with the IM)

**Hypoxia**

If a patient is irritable, anxious, or somnolent, suspect hypoxia until proven otherwise. Most common etiologies include *opioid overdose, silent MI, aspiration,* and *new onset ARDS.* Hypoxia can be a precursor to a *serious* chain of events during which a patient may become moribund. Involve your chief resident early in this scenario.

*Diagnosis*

- Oxygen saturation monitor to bedside
- ABG
- CBC, electrolytes ($Ca^{2+}$, $Mg^{2+}$, $K^+$)
- CXR portable
- ECG, cardiac enzymes

*Treatment*

- Apply supplemental $O_2$, 4-L nasal cannula and advance as appropriate.
- If patient still hypoxic on 6-L $O_2$ nasal cannula, discuss transferring patient to the ICU with your chief resident.
- Naloxone (Narcan) 0.4–2 mg IV q3min prn opioid overdose.
- Flumazenil (Romazicon) 0.2 mg IV q1min (may repeat × 4) prn benzodiazepine overdose.

# 16

# Head and Neck

**Neck Mass**

- 99.9% of neck masses are benign.
- Inflammation is the most common cause with lymphadenitis the most common diagnosis.
- Congenital masses include thyroglossal duct cyst, branchial cleft cyst, and lymphangioma (cystic hygroma).
- Differential diagnosis of malignant neck masses: lymphoma, squamous cell carcinoma rhabdomyosarcoma, fibrosarcoma, thyroid cancer, neuroblastoma.

**Neck Masses in Adults**

*Statistics*

- 85% of nonthyroid neck masses in adults are malignant.
- 80% of malignant neck masses are metastatic, mostly from primaries originating *above* the clavicle.
- If a patient is >40 years old, a neck mass should be considered malignant until proven otherwise; especially if history of tobacco or alcohol consumption or history of radiation exposure.

---

**FACT BOX 37**

- Most common cancers presenting as a neck mass in children: lymphoma (50%), sarcoma, and medullary thyroid carcinoma
- Most common cancers presenting as a neck mass in adults: squamous cell carcinoma from head/neck primary, malignant melanoma

## Assessment—ABCs: Is There an Impending Airway Obstruction?

### Differential Diagnosis

- Congenital (thyroglossal duct cyst, branchial cleft cyst)
- Benign neoplasm
- Infectious (lymphadenopathy)
- Malignant (cancer of salivary gland, thyroid cancer, lymphoma, leukemia)
- Metastatic disease (from skin, thyroid, head and neck, lung, breast, GI, or GU primary)

### History

- Age is an important factor
  - 20s and 30s—papillary thyroid cancer, lymphoma, leukemia
  - >40—metastatic cancer from lung, breast, oropharynx
- Tobacco use (smoking)
- EtOH

---

**FACT BOX 38**

Good rule of thumb is to ask:
How long has the mass been there?
- 7 days—Inflammation
- 7 months—Cancer
- 7 years—Congenital or benign

- Radiation exposure
- Family history

*Symptoms*

- Mass
- Pain
- Airway obstruction, stridor
- Bleeding
- Fever, weight loss, night sweats (constitutional symptoms)
- Recurrent infectious illness (upper respiratory infection [URI], otitis)
- Dysphagia, odynophagia
- Hoarse voice (impingement on recurrent laryngeal nerve)

*Physical Exam*

Include a thorough examination of the scalp, eyes, ears, nose, mouth, teeth, gums, tongue (palpate with gloved finger), hypopharynx, nasopharynx, and larynx (mirror or scope). Does the mass move with swallowing? If yes, think thyroid; if no, probably not thyroid.

### Location of the Mass

*Malignant*

- Midline—Likely to be related to the thyroid
- Supraclavicular—Likely to be from a primary tumor below the clavicle
- Posterior Triangle—Metastatic disease from the nasopharynx
- Submandibular—From oral cavity or anterior 2/3 of the tongue

*Benign*

- Anterior Midline—Suggests aberrant thyroid, thyroglossal cyst, pyramidal lobe, 1st branchial cleft cyst, teratoma, abscess, or aneurysm of aortic arch
- Anterior Lateral—2nd branchial cleft cyst, torticollis, thyroid mass, carotid artery mass

- Mid-Lateral—Suggests cystic hygroma, lymphangiocele
- Posterior Triangle—Suggests adenopathy

*Laboratory Evaluation*

CBC with differential, thyroid function tests, PPD, Monospot

*Radiographic Workup*

Goal is to identify the primary tumor
- Plain Films—Chest x-ray, lateral soft tissue neck films, sinus films
- CT scan of head, neck, chest, and abdomen—With and without contrast
- Radioisotope Scan—Thyroid scan w/$I^{125}$

If primary tumor not found, secondary workup includes:
- Pan-endoscopy (laryngoscopy, esophagoscopy, bronchoscopy, and nasopharyngoscopy) looking for mucosal lesions
- Random biopsies (if the endoscopic exam is negative) of the nasopharynx, tonsils, base of the tongue, and pyriform sinus (common site of laryngeal cancer)
- Open biopsy of the neck mass—If all radiologic studies, endoscopies, and mucosa biopsies are negative

*Treatment*

If primary cancer is confirmed by biopsy, the metastatic neck disease is treated in conjunction with the primary tumor.
- Radical Neck Dissection—The sternocleidomastoid (SCM) muscle, internal jugular vein, spinal accessory nerve, and all cervical lymphatics are removed from the affected side. Indicated to treat metastatic squamous cell carcinoma with an unknown primary or in conjunction with resection of a known primary.
- Modified Radical Neck Dissection—Same as the radical but spares the spinal accessory nerve.
- Modified Neck Dissection—Remove cervical lymphatics, spare the SCM muscle, internal jugular vein, and spinal accessory nerve. *Indicated for:*

    ○ Elective neck dissections
    ○ Single node <3 cm that is to be treated with postop XRT
    ○ Differentiated thyroid cancers with neck metastasis
    ○ Simultaneous bilateral neck dissections
    ○ Examples include: supra-omohyoid, anterior triangle, posterior triangle.
- Radiation therapy alone for many early lesions.
- Postop radiation therapy and chemotherapy for advanced lesions.
- New advances in organ-sparing protocols use radiation therapy and chemotherapy as primary treatments without resection of primary tumor.

**Thyroid Nodule**

*Anatomy*

*Arteries*

- Superior thyroid artery is the first branch off the external carotid artery.
- Inferior thyroid artery arises from thyrocervical trunk off the subclavian artery.
- Thyroid artery occasionally arises from the aortic arch.

*Nerves*

- Left recurrent laryngeal nerve loops around the arch of the aorta.
- Right recurrent laryngeal nerve loops around the subclavian artery.
- Damage to a single recurrent laryngeal nerve leads to loss of voice.
- Damage to both recurrent laryngeal nerves may cause occlusion of airway by vocal cord apposition. Tracheostomy is indicated.
- Damage to the external branch of the superior laryngeal nerve leads to loss of singing voice.

*History*

- Head and neck radiation
- Radiation exposure of any kind
- Family history of "neck" cancers (MEN syndromes)

*Physical Exam*

Findings on thyroid exam suggestive of malignancy:
- Firm nodule
- Solitary nodule (20% of solitary nodules are malignant)
- Ipsilateral nodal enlargement

---

**FACT BOX 39**

20% of cold nodules will be malignant.

---

*Laboratory Evaluation*

Thyroid function tests (TFT) are usually of little value because <1% of thyroid tumors are hyperfunctioning.

### Diagnostic Studies

- Radioisotope (iodine technetium) scan—Cold nodule is malignant 20% of the time, but as many as 40% of thyroid cancers will be hot.
- Laryngoscopy may identify ipsilateral vocal cord paralysis.
- Biopsy—Many different approaches can be used and usually depend on the pathologist who will eventually identify the specimen.
  - *Core needle biopsy*—Provides tissue for histologic examination. Easiest for pathologist to interpret, but most difficult for patient to tolerate. Best for large nodules (>3 cm diameter).
  - *Fine needle aspiration (FNA)*—Provides cells for cytologic examination. Least invasive for the patients, but most difficult for pathologist to distinguish between benign or malignant follicular neoplasms. FNA has a 1%–10% false negative and a 0%–2% false positive rate in the most experienced hands.

○ *Surgical Excisional Biopsy*—Thyroid lobectomy with frozen section biopsy of significant nodes. The remaining management is based on the results of the frozen section.

### Pathology

*Papillary*

- 80% of all thyroid cancers
- History of radiation exposure
- Spread to lymphatics
- Associated with psammoma bodies
- 90% 20-year survival

*Follicular*

- 20% of thyroid cancers
- Hematogenous spread
- 80% 20-year survival if no vascular invasion (20% survival with vascular invasion)

*Medullary*

- <10% of thyroid cancer
- Arise from C-cells of thyroid and have elevations in calcitonin
- Associated with MEN II
- Lymphatic spread
- 50% 20-year survival for stage I, 10% for stage II

*Anaplastic*

- <10% of thyroid cancer
- Worst prognosis

---

**FACT BOX 40**

Family members of any patient with medullary thyroid cancer should be screened for MEN II with calcitonin, PTH, urinary catecholamines.

---

## *Management*

- Benign—No more therapy
- Papillary neoplasm <1.5 cm diameter with negative nodes—No more therapy
- Papillary or other type >1.5 cm—Near total thyroidectomy with postop radioiodine ablation
- Medullary Thyroid Cancer—Total thyroidectomy and mid-neck lymph node dissection
- Anaplastic Tumors—Extremely aggressive, usually metastatic at time of diagnosis. Extremely difficult to resect. Should be treated with radiation and chemotherapy for palliation.

### *Adjuvant Therapy*

- All patients with cancer get postop radioiodine ablation whether they had a total thyroidectomy or lobectomy.
- Residual thyroid tissue can show up on iodine scan.
- All patients get Synthroid for life to suppress TSH.

# 17

# Breast Disease

*Statistics*

- 12% (1 in 9) of women will develop breast cancer in their lifetime. 3.5% will die of the disease.
- More than half of all women with breast cancer are over age 65.
- <5% of breast cancers are associated with genetic predisposition.
- Fibroadenoma is the most common breast mass in women <30 years old.
- Fibrocystic change is the most common breast pathology in women <40 years old.

*Anatomy*

Axillary lymph nodes are divided into three levels:
- I—Lateral to the pectoralis minor
- II—Deep to the pectoralis minor
- III—Medial to the pectoralis minor

*Relevant Nerves*
- *Intercostal Brachial Nerve*—Provides sensation to the skin of the upper medial arm. Transverses the axilla after exiting the chest wall at the third interspace.
- *Long Thoracic Nerve (of Bell)*—From cervical roots 5–7, courses close to the chest wall to supply the serratus anterior muscle. Damage results in winged scapula.

- *Thoracodorsal Nerve*—Follows the long thoracic artery and vein along the lateral border of the axilla to innervate the latissimus dorsi.
- *Lateral Pectoral Nerve*—From the lateral cord of the brachial plexus, innervates both the pectoralis major and minor.

## Benign Breast Disease

### Fibrocystic Change

A common disorder characterized by tender cystic or nodular lesions of the breast. Possibly represents an exaggerated response of breast parenchyma to circulating hormones. Affects women 20–40 years of age and usually resolves with decreasing hormones associated with menopause. Also known as cystic mastopathy.

### Symptoms and Physical Findings

- Pain, swelling, and tenderness.
- Focal areas of nodularity, induration, or cysts.
- Symptoms are usually bilateral.
- Fluctuate with the menstrual cycle.
- May produce multiple duct discharge from the nipple.

### Diagnosis

- History and physical exam sufficient in most cases.
- Ultrasound if symptoms severe, persistent, or if on specific area of the breast worrisome.
- Ultrasound-guided FNA if cyst(s) identified. If cyst is benign, the aspirate will not be bloody and ultrasound will reveal that the cyst has resolved. If cyst fails to resolve or if aspirate is bloody or equivocal, further workup for cancer should be done (ultrasound-guided FNA of breast cysts also has therapeutic effects by relieving pressure and discomfort).

### Management of Fibrocystic Change

- Monthly breast self-exam by the patient; annual breast exam by a physician

- Baseline mammogram at age 35 and annual mammography starting at age 40
- Avoidance of xanthine (tea, coffee, chocolate) and nicotine
- Danazol 50–200 mg po bid for severe symptoms
- Tamoxifen 20 mg po qd for 4–6 weeks for patients with severe incapacitating symptoms
- Vitamin E 400 IU po qd for mild to moderate symptoms

### Fibroadenoma

Most common breast mass in women under the age of 30.

#### Symptoms and Physical Findings

- Presents as a painless solitary breast mass usually found by the patient on self-examination
- Well-circumscribed firm rubbery mass 1–5 cm in diameter
- Solitary but can be bilateral
- May increase in size with oral contraceptive use or cyclically with menses

#### Diagnosis

- Mammogram may be negative or may demonstrate a benign appearing mass
- Ultrasound identifies a well-circumscribed solid lesion. Excisional biopsy indicated if distressing to the patient or if dynamic in nature (if any change in the lesion).

#### Management

- Conservative therapy with close follow-up of a static lesion in a young patient acceptable
- Excisional biopsy if lesion changes or if patient anxious

---

**FACT BOX 41**

Intraductal papilloma is the most common cause of bloody nipple discharge.

---

### Intraductal Papilloma

A benign solitary lesion that presents as a bloody single duct nipple discharge. Discharge fluid should by evaluated for cytology.

#### Symptoms and Physical Findings

• Nipple discharge emanates from a single duct. Usually no mass is palpated and mammogram is negative.

#### Diagnosis

• Ductogram—Radiocontrast is injected into the duct to evaluate for any masses or lesions.
• Biopsy by injecting sterile methylene blue into the affected duct. Excision of all blue stained breast tissue follows.

#### Management of Intraductal Papilloma

• Excisional biopsy is indicated as there is approximately a 5% chance of occult cancer.
• No further treatment after biopsy if benign.

## Malignant Breast Disease

### Terminology

Carcinoma—Cancerous proliferation of epithelial cells lining ducts (ductal carcinoma) and lobules (lobular carcinoma)

Sarcoma—Cancerous proliferation of the cells of the supporting stroma

Carcinoma in Situ—Cancerous proliferation has not yet penetrated the basement membrane; associated with zero risk of metastases.

Invasive Carcinoma—Cancer that has invaded the basement membrane

### Ductal Carcinoma in Situ (DCIS)

DCIS is also known as intraductal carcinoma or carcinoma of lactiferous duct epithelium with no invasion of the basement membrane.

*Symptoms and Physical Findings*

- Most found incidentally on mammography
- Few present with palpable mass

*Diagnosis*

- Need tissue for histological diagnosis.
- Pathologist must carefully analyze the specimen for evidence of invasion of basement membrane.

*Management of DCIS*

- Partial mastectomy with negative margins
- Postoperative radiation therapy if >1 cm

**Lobular Carcinoma in Situ (LCIS)**

Carcinoma in situ of epithelium of breast lobules (acini). Also known as lobular neoplasia. 20% of patients will develop breast cancer in either the ipsilateral or contralateral breast within 20 years.

---

FACT BOX **42**

LCIS is NOT cancer; however, it is a predictor of future cancer in either breast (most commonly infiltrating ductal cancer).
Negative margins are not necessary in LCIS (it is not cancer).

---

*Symptoms and Physical Findings*

- Never forms a palpable mass
- Has no mammographic characteristics
- Usually found incidentally after biopsy for other reasons

*Diagnosis*

- Incidental finding on breast biopsy

*Management of LCIS*

- Observation with yearly mammogram and physical exam
- Prophylactic bilateral mastectomy—if patient has significant family history of breast cancer
- Bilateral oophorectomy

### Infiltrating Ductal Carcinoma

Carcinoma of lactiferous duct epithelium that has invaded through the basement membrane into the surrounding stroma.

*Symptoms and Physical Findings*

- Breast lump found on physical exam represents the majority of cases.
- Microcalcifications are often seen on mammogram.

*Diagnosis*

- Mammogram to assess for multifocal disease.
- FNA (with or without US guidance)—performed with a 20-G–21-G syringe (15% false negative results).
- Core Needle Biopsy—obtains more tissue and is more accurate than FNA.
- Excisional biopsy—removes entire mass with negative margins.
- Wire localization biopsy—a wire in inserted under fluoroscopy into an area of microcalcifications. The wire and surrounding tissue are then surgically removed. Confirmation of complete excision is done by x-ray of specimen (microcalcifications present in specimen).

*Management of Infiltrating Ductal Carcinoma*

There are four main operations for breast cancer.
- Partial mastectomy with radiation therapy
- Partial mastectomy with axillary lymph node dissection
- Modified radical mastectomy
- Modified radical mastectomy with TRAM flap reconstruction

### *Invasive Lobular Carcinoma*

Carcinoma of the breast acini that invades the basement membrane.

*Symptoms and Physical Findings*

- Breast mass most common finding
- Mammographic lesion

*Diagnosis*

- Histologic examination of tissue (*see Infiltrating ductal carcinoma*)

*Management of Invasive Lobular Carcinoma*

- Same as infiltrating ductal carcinoma

## The Patient with Breast Cancer

### *Historical Facts That Increase the Risk of Breast Cancer*

- Family history
- History of chronic cystic mastitis
- History of contralateral breast cancer
- Nulliparity
- Early menarche
- Late menopause

### *Findings on Physical Exam Suggestive of Cancer*

- Breast lump is the presenting symptom of breast cancer in 85%–90% of women.
- Hard mass.
- Unilateral breast enlargement.
- Skin dimpling.
- Redness.
- Spontaneous nipple discharge or edema.
- Painless mass.
- Lymph nodes (axillary and supra- and infraclavicular) that are enlarged, firm, fixed, or painless suggest cancer.

### Laboratory Evaluation

- None initially. If mass proves to be cancer, a staging workup will be required.

### Radiographic Evaluation

- Mammogram to assess any palpable lesion for microcalcifications and to determine whether additional foci of microcalcification are present in either breast (i.e., to determine the presence of synchronous or metastatic disease). There is a 15% false negative rate.
- Ultrasound may be useful to differentiate cystic from solid mass.

### Diagnosis

- Diagnosis is made with tissue biopsy. Sample is obtained in several fashions: core needle, incisional, or excisional biopsy. Excisional biopsy is generally the best course.
- Stereotactic excisional biopsy can be performed on radiographically identifiable lesions with only a 5-mm incision.

### Differential Diagnosis of Breast Carcinoma

- Ductal carcinoma in situ
- Lobular carcinoma in situ
- Infiltrating ductal carcinoma
- Invasive lobular carcinoma
- Inflammatory breast carcinoma
- Paget's disease of the nipple

### Staging of Breast Cancer

Breast cancer metastasizes to liver, lung, bone, and brain. Complete staging will evaluate each of these areas.

#### Initial Evaluation

Complete physical exam will determine if there are any mental status changes or bone pain that would require CT of head and bone scan.

- Liver function test (if abnormal CT scan of abdomen)
- Chest x-ray
- Serum $Ca^{2+}$

---

**FACT BOX 43**

Many cancers follow the same pattern. Once a tissue diagnosis is made, a staging workup is required. This is usually physical exam, liver function test, CXR, serum calcium.

---

### *Treatment of Breast Cancer*

*Surgery*

*Modified Radical Mastectomy*—Surgical resection of all breast tissue with complete axillary node dissection.

*Partial Mastectomy*—Wide local excision of the tumor with 1-cm margins. Conserves the remainder of the breast tissue. Requires 4500 centiGray of radiation therapy to the breast for local control.

*Partial Mastectomy with Axillary Lymph Node Dissection*—Remove levels I and II lymph nodes of the axilla. Goals of axillary lymph node dissection are to stage the tumor and to remove gross disease.

*Sentinel Node Biopsy*—Radiolabeled colloid and blue dye are injected into the breast tissue. These subsequently move through the lymphatics to the first draining axillary lymph node (sentinel node). The sentinel node is excised and evaluated with multiple sections. If tumor cells are present in this node it suggests that the primary has metastasized to the axilla. If it is negative it suggests that the cancer is contained within the breast. This technique may, in the future, eliminate the need to perform a formal axillary lymph node dissection minimizing the associated morbidity. There are currently several clinical trials evaluating sentinel lymph node biopsy versus formal axillary node dissection.

*Adjuvant Therapy*

- XRT is for local control where chemotherapy is for systemic control (metastasis).
- Common chemotherapy agents—CMF-cyclophosphamide, methotrexate, 5-fluorouracil.
- Pre- or postmenopausal women with negative node >1-cm tumor.
- Any patient with positive nodes.

*Hormonal Therapy*

- Use antiestrogen drugs such as tamoxifen to prevent recurrence, improve long-term survival.
- Most beneficial for ER/PR positive tumors.
- Pre- or postmenopausal.
- Node positive.
- High-risk node-negative (>1 cm).

---

**FACT BOX 44**

**Clinical Study**

NSABP-B06 found no difference in survival between MRM and partial mastectomy with or without XRT. Partial mastectomy alone is associated with a decreased disease-free survival.

---

# 18

# Cardiovascular

**Coronary Artery Disease**

*Etiology*

- Arteriosclerosis

---

**FACT BOX 45**

Aspirin is the most significant postop drug to help maintain graft and coronary artery patency (anyone suspected of having an MI should immediately receive ASA 325 mg chewed)

---

*Important Risk Factors*

- Male sex
- Family history of coronary artery disease
- Smoking
- Hypercholesterolemia, obesity
- Diabetes
- Hypertension (HTN)
- Peripheral vascular disease
- Sedentary lifestyle
- Diet rich in saturated fats

### Diagnosis

- ECG—May demonstrate acute ischemia or old infarction
- Cardiac Enzymes—If increased, are diagnostic of acute infarction
  - CK-MB
  - Troponin (early rise)
- Stress Test—Used to uncover inducible ischemia
- Stress Thallium—Used to diagnose areas of ischemia or areas of old infarction
- Cardiac Catheterization—Invasive contrast study to evaluate coronary anatomy
- Echocardiogram (ECHO)

### Indications for Coronary Artery Bypass Grafting (CABG)

- Triple-vessel disease
- Refractory postinfarction angina
- Left main disease
- Angioplasty failure
- ECG changes consistent with MI and ischemia

### Cardiac Vasculature

Coronary vessels most commonly occluded. The occlusion must be proximal to be amenable to bypass.
- LAD (left anterior descending)
- LCx (left circumflex)
- RCA (right coronary artery)
- Marginal artery

### Treatment

#### Coronary Artery Bypass Grafting (CABG)

Bypass of occluded segment with internal mammary artery (IMA) and/or saphenous vein grafts
- Six bypasses possible.
- Left IMA has 10-year patency of 80%–90%.

- Saphenous vein has 10-year patency of 50%.
- Alternative grafts: Radial and gastroepiploic artery.

There is significant improvement in perfusion with triple-vessel disease following coronary artery bypass.

# 19

# Thoracic Tumors

**Solitary Pulmonary Nodule**

*Statistics*

- Lung cancer is the leading cause of cancer deaths in the United States.
- 10% of solitary pulmonary nodules are malignant, 80% if >50 years old.
- 85%–90% of malignant nodules are bronchogenic cancer.
- 95% of patients with lung cancer are over 40 years of age.
- 50% of patients are unresectable at initial diagnosis.
- Overall prognosis for nodule found to be malignant: 40%–60% 5-year survival (however, nodules <2 cm may be associated with 80% 5-year survival).

*History*

The three most significant factors suggesting a malignant process are:
- Smoking history
- Age >50 years old
- Change in chronic cough

---

**FACT BOX 46**

Over 40 carcinogens have been identified in cigarette smoke. However, only 20% of smokers develop lung cancer.

---

Other important factors include:

- Anorexia
- Weight loss
- Fever
- Chills

### *Radiology: CXR*

- Previous CXR for a comparison is extremely helpful.
- If a lesion shows no change in size over 2 years, it is probably benign (mean doubling time for malignant pulmonary nodule is 4 months).
- Calcification is usually a sign of a benign lesion.
- If an old film is not available or if new or growing lesion is identified, additional radiologic evaluation with CT may be required. CT may detect calcifications or other nodules not seen on CXR.

### *Diagnosis*

*Needle Aspiration*—Diagnostic accuracy of 85%–90%. Most accurate for lesions that are peripheral and are greater than 2 cm in diameter. Risk of pneumothorax is 30%.

*Fiberoptic Bronchoscopy*—Used to obtain brushings and washings. Diagnostic accuracy of 90% for endobronchial lesions, but only 60% for parenchymal lesions. Lower risk associated with this procedure. Useful in staging the cancer.

*VATS* (Video-Assisted Thoracoscopic Surgery)

*Thoracotomy with Wedge Resection or Lobectomy*—This is the most direct means for establishing a diagnosis. It can also serve as definitive treatment for a cure.

*Observation*—Best way to make a definitive diagnosis:

- A lesion is considered benign only if another diagnosis is made to describe the pathology.
- Observation is never satisfactory for a smoker over 40 years of age.

### *Differential Diagnosis*

- Primary lung malignancy

- Pulmonary metastasis from a distant primary (e.g., breast, testicular)
- Benign tumor (hamartoma, hemangioma)
- Infection (fungal, bacterial, tuberculosis, hydatid cyst, coccidioidomycosis)
- Foreign body pneumonitis (lipid pneumonia, pneumoconiosis, talc granulomas, amyloidosis, aspiration pneumonia)
- Vascular (pulmonary infarction, hemorrhage, hemosiderosis)
- Rheumatologic (rheumatoid nodule, Wegener's granulomatosis)

## Lung Cancer

Usually subdivided bases on histologic type:

### *Non–Small Cell Carcinoma*

- *Adenocarcinoma* is the most common lung cancer (45%). Arises in peripheral lung parenchyma.
- *Squamous cell carcinoma* is strongly associated with smoking and arises from metaplasia of tracheobronchial tree. Usually more proximal in location.
- *Large cell carcinoma* is rare and is located either centrally or peripherally. Has the poorest prognosis.

### *Small Cell Carcinoma*

Worse prognosis and not usually amenable to surgical resection.
- *Small cell carcinoma* is usually centrally located and neurosecretory in nature. Chemotherapy is primary treatment.

### *When Not to Operate*

Surgical resection is not curative and therefore is contraindicated in cases of:
- Extensive ipsilateral node involvement (N2) (paratracheal or subcarinal nodes)
- Contralateral nodes (N3)
- Distant metastasis (M1)
- Malignant pleural effusion
- Superior vena cava syndrome

- Recurrent laryngeal nerve involvement
- Phrenic nerve paralysis

---

**FACT BOX 47**

Patients with a predicted postop FEV$_1$ >800 or 2.0 L preop can usually tolerate lung resection.

---

## Mediastinal Disease

### Anterior

- Thymomas
- Teratomas
- Lymphomas
- Germ cell tumors

### Middle

- Pericardial cysts
- Bronchogenic cysts
- Ascending aortic aneurysm

### Posterior

- Neuroblastomas
- Pheochromocytomas

# 20

# Hemoptysis

**Hemoptysis**

Patients with chronic bronchitis may produce faintly blood-tinged sputum from time to time, but all other cases of hemoptysis deserve a thorough workup.

*History*

- Onset
- Associated findings
- Color of the blood (bright red blood indicative of active hemorrhage)
- Whether clotted or not
- History of trauma

*Labs*

- CBC and coagulation profile (PT/PTT), T&C

---

**FACT BOX 48**

In a patient who is actively bleeding, always obtain:
- CBC
- PT/pTT
- T&C

---

## Radiology

- CXR to assess for old or new inflammatory lesions, masses, malignancies, vascular abnormalities

## Diagnosis

*Fiberoptic Bronchoscopy*—Virtually every patient should undergo bronchoscopy. Goal is to determine the site of the bleeding or at least the correct bronchus.

## Management

- Most bleeding stops by itself.
- The massively bleeding patient should lie with the bleeding lung down (dependent).
- If bleeding continues an endotracheal tube can be placed in the right mainstem bronchus to keep the blood confined to one lung.
- Definitive treatment involves surgical resection of localized lesions such as bronchial adenomas or pulmonary sequestrations.
- Generalized diseases such as widespread bronchiectasis are left alone.
- For uncontrollable bleeding, lobectomy or pneumonectomy may be required.

## Differential Diagnosis

- Arteriovenous (AV) malformation
- Bronchogenic cancer
- Bronchiectasis
- Idiopathic
- TB
- Atypical mycobacteria
- Infections (pneumonia, abscess, fungal)
- Miscellaneous (pulmonary fibrosis, coagulopathy, CHF, sarcoid)

# 21

# Gastrointestinal System

## Abdominal Surgical Maneuvers

*Pringle Maneuver*—Occlusion of the porta hepatis (hepatic artery and portal vein) to decrease blood flow to the liver

*Kocher Maneuver*—Transection of the lateral peritoneal attachments of duodenum to allow medial retraction

*Cattel Maneuver*—Mobilization of the ascending colon to midline to allow medial retraction of the entire right colon

*Mattox Maneuver*—Mobilization of the descending colon to midline to allow medial retraction of the entire left colon

## Abdominal Anatomy

*White Line of Hilton*—Between the external and internal anal sphincters

*Space of Rolan*—An avascular area in the mesentery to the left of the middle colic artery

*Jackson's Veils*—Peritoneal folds across the ascending colon from the cecum to the right hepatic flexure

*Treves' Folds*—Avascular ileocecal peritoneal folds

*Sudeck's Point*—Watershed area between the superior hemorrhoidal and middle hemorrhoidal arteries

*Griffith Point*—Watershed area between the midgut and hindgut blood supply in the transverse colon

*White Line of Toldt*—The lateral peritoneal attachment of the colon

# 22

# Acute Abdomen

## Most Common and Quick Facts

- Most common site of perforation in the colon is the cecum.
- Bloody diarrhea with progressive severe abdominal pain suggests colonic ischemia.
- Adhesions are the most common cause of small bowel obstruction.
- Patients with common bile duct or kidney stones cannot find a comfortable position.
- Pain from acute peptic ulcer disease is usually relieved by food and antacids.
- Pain is worsened by food in acute cholecystitis and/or pancreatitis.
- Acute gastric dilatation can cause hypotension secondary to reflex vagal discharge.
- Air fluid levels in the small intestine are abnormal and may be secondary to paralytic ileus or obstruction.
- Initial treatment of sigmoid volvulus is with sigmoidscopy and decompression.
- Thumbprinting of the bowel wall seen on x-ray may indicate ischemic or gangrenous bowel.
- Boerhaave's syndrome is esophageal rupture secondary to violent vomiting.
- Gastrografin (diatrizoate meglumine) is an $H_2O$ soluble contrast medium used if bowel perforation is suspected.

## History

Ask patients with abdominal pain about location, character, onset, duration, aggravating and alleviating factors, and associated symptoms.

*Perforated Viscus*—Sharp, sudden, severe pain that awakens patient from sleep

*Bowel Obstruction*—Intermittent crampy pain

*Strangulated Bowel*—Dull constant pain

*Acute Cholecystitis*—RUQ pain that radiates to the posterior right costal margin, scapula, and shoulder

*Acute Pancreatitis*—Epigastric pain that radiates to the back

*Ureteral Colic*—Flank pain that radiates to the testicle if high in the urethra or to the perineum if at the ureterovesical junction

*Acute Appendicitis*—Crampy abdominal pain that originates at the umbilicus and moves to the RLQ as a continuous sharp pain

*Ectopic Pregnancy*—Unilateral crampy abdominal pain, sharp stabbing if ruptured, amenorrhea or abnormal bleeding

*Pelvic Inflammatory Disease*—Bilateral lower abdominal pain, constant or dull, associated with fever, chills, and vaginal discharge

## Associated Symptoms

*Vomiting*—May result from the severity of the pain or from the intra-abdominal pathology itself. Clear vomitus suggests an obstructed pylorus. Bile-stained vomitus suggests an obstruction distal to the common bile duct.

*Anorexia*—Usually the result of the pain, but in appendicitis often precedes the pain.

*Constipation, Diarrhea, or Change in Bowel Habit*—Failure to pass flatus associated with cramping abdominal pain and vomiting supports the diagnosis of mechanical bowel obstruction.

*Menstrual*—History and contraceptive use.

## Past Medical History to Ask About

- Previous surgery (appendectomy, cholecystectomy, gastric or intestinal surgery)

120

- History of inguinal or abdominal hernia
- Sickle cell disease

---

**FACT BOX 49**

Nonsurgical causes of acute abdominal pain:
- Pneumonia
- MI
- DKA
- Hepatitis
- Musculoskeletal

---

**Physical Exam**

- General Appearance—Ability to answer questions, position in bed, degree of obvious pain or discomfort
- Abdomen—inspect, auscultate, percuss, and palpate
  - Inspection (scars, hernias, obvious masses, abdominal wall, defects, distention)
  - Auscultation (frequency and pitch of bowel sounds)
  - Percussion (tympani, gas, fluid)
  - Palpation (rebound, guarding, voluntary guarding, masses)
- Pelvic—Cervical discharge, vaginal bleeding, cervical motion tenderness, uterine or adnexal tenderness
- Rectal—Pelvic tenderness, mass, perirectal abscess, Hemoccult the stool

**Labs**

- CBC, Chem-18 (LFT), UA, amylase, bHCG

**Radiology**

- Abdominal Films (supine and erect)—Look for free air from perforated viscus or air fluid levels from obstruction.
- Ultrasound to evaluate gallbladder, liver, spleen, pancreas, kidney, and aorta.

- CT scan of abdomen.
- Arteriography.

## Differential Diagnosis in the Acute Abdomen

*Perforated Peptic Ulcer*—Usually from a duodenal ulcer, common in men 40–50 years of age. Pain is sudden in onset and severe and is located first in the epigastrium and then becomes generalized. Shoulder pain is common and suggests diaphragmatic irritation. Patient usually lies very still in the supine position. The abdomen is rigid. Bowel sounds are hypoactive or absent. There is an elevated WBC (12–20 K) with a left shift. Serum amylase may be elevated. Free air is seen under the diaphragm on x-ray in 75% of cases.

*Acute Cholecystitis*—Most commonly occurs in women 30–60 years of age. The ache begins as a constant dull ache in the RUQ and epigastric area. Patients move about in order to relieve the pain and appear restless. The abdomen may be distended. Bowel sounds are hypoactive. Tenderness is maximal in the RUQ especially on inspiration (*Murphy's sign*: splinting on a deep inspiration due to pain). A normal or mildly elevated WBC count is usual. An elevated bilirubin of 2–2.5 may occur, but a bilirubin over 3 suggests common duct stones. Ultrasound can assess the diameter of the biliary tree, the presence of stones, the appearance of the gallbladder wall and its contents. HIDA (hepatobiliary iododiacetic acid) scan shows nonvisualization of the gallbladder if the cystic duct is occluded.

*Acute Pancreatitis*—May present with sudden severe onset of epigastric pain radiating to the back. Anorexia, nausea, and vomiting are common and the vomiting does not provide relief. Abdominal tenderness is present in the epigastrium. Bowel sounds are hypoactive or absent. WBC count is usually elevated (12–22 K). Amylase and lipase are elevated within a few hours of onset. Plain films are nondiagnostic. CT and ultrasound are used to diagnose complications.

*Chronic Pancreatitis*—Differs in that there are previous episodes of the pain and it becomes constant. There are frequently pancreatic calcifications on x-ray. Amylase and lipase may only be mildly elevated.

*Acute Appendicitis*—Abdominal pain begins about the umbilicus and finally to the RLQ. Anorexia, nausea, and vomiting are common. Pain precedes nausea and vomiting. After localization of the pain to the RLQ, there is RLQ tenderness and peritoneal signs (rebound, obturator sign, Rovsing's sign). Guarding occurs when there is localized peritonitis. WBC is usually elevated. Plain films are usually normal, although a fecalith may be seen (5% of cases). Ultrasound and CT can be helpful, especially in children, the elderly, or obese patients.

*Pelvic Inflammatory Disease (Acute Salpingitis)*—Usually seen in women before menopause. It causes pelvic pain in the RLQ and/or LLQ. It often becomes symptomatic just following the menstrual period. The pain is rarely associated with anorexia, nausea, vomiting. The pain is usually bilateral and associated with low-grade fever. There is tenderness of both lower quadrants and with movement of the cervix (cervical motion tenderness). There are frequently adnexal masses with an associated vaginal discharge.

*Ovarian Cysts*—May present as an acute abdomen if torsion occurs: sudden onset of severe pain in one side of the lower abdomen. Pelvic exam may reveal a palpable mass.

*Ectopic Pregnancy*—Tubal pregnancy may present with sudden lower abdominal pain that is sharp and persistent, with or without nausea and vomiting. Patient may give a history of a missed or scant menstrual period. Diagnosis is established by a positive HCG and determining if there is an intrauterine pregnancy via ultrasound.

*Renal Calculi*—May cause severe abdominal or flank pain. As the stone descends into the ureter, the pain may radiate to the groin, testicle, or perineum. The pain is sudden and excruciating and may wax and wane. Supine abdominal films and IVP should be obtained (90% of stones are radiopaque). Spinal CT scan is replacing IVP at many centers.

*Meckel's Diverticulum*—This is a persistence of the vitelline duct on the antimesenteric border of the distal ileum that produces bleeding, obstruction, and less commonly acute abdominal pain from diverticulitis. Meckel's diverticulitis is difficult to differentiate from acute appendicitis.

> **FACT BOX 50**
>
> Meckel's rule of 2's: 2 feet from ileocecal valve, 2% of population, 2% symptomatic.

*Acute Diverticulitis*—May result from congenital or acquired (most common) colonic diverticula, usually involving the sigmoid colon. Occurs more in older patients. Presents with LLQ pain, chills, and fever. Vomiting and anorexia are uncommon. The abdomen is slightly distended and the LLQ is tender to palpation. A mass may be palpable just medial to the anterior superior iliac spine. Diagnosis confirmed on CT scan of the abdomen and pelvis.

*Acute Small Bowel Obstruction (SBO)*—The first symptom is sudden, sharp, colicky periumbilical abdominal pain that is crampy in nature. Between episodes of colic, the patient may be asymptomatic. Nausea and vomiting occur early, and emesis may temporarily relieve the pain. The color of the vomitus is first green then changes to yellow brown color with feculent odor. Auscultation reveals high-pitched hyperactive bowel sounds. WBC count is elevated in the 12–20 K range. If the obstruction is in the mid- or distal small bowel, the abdominal films show dilated loops of small bowel with air–fluid levels. The nonobstructed colon is devoid of gas and feces.

> **FACT BOX 51**
>
> Major causes of SBO are:
> - Adhesions
> - Hernia
> - Tumor

*Acute Large Bowel Obstruction*—This occurs more frequently in patients over 40 years of age, is gradual in onset, and presents with constipation, obstipation, and abdominal distention. The abdomen is tympanic to percussion and is minimally tender to palpation. On x-ray, the large bowel may be distended if the ileocecal valve is competent. Major causes include tumor, diverticulitis, and volvulus.

*Volvulus*—Sigmoid volvulus is the most common and occurs in older patients. Diagnosis is established by supine and upright abdominal films and water-soluble contrast enema (Gastrografin). Cecal volvulus occurs in middle-aged and older patients and presents as sudden onset of cramping RLQ and epigastric pain associated with nausea and vomiting. Diagnosis is established by abdominal films showing a dilated cecum and ascending colon.

## Indications for Abdominal Operation

- Any patient with acute abdominal pain lasting longer than 6 hours
- Abdominal rigidity
- Increasing tenderness locally
- Progressive abdominal distention
- Abdominal pain associated with shock
- Abdominal pain associated with septicemia (leukocytosis >20 K)
- Laboratory findings consistent with gut ischemia (increasing lactate, metabolic acidosis)
- Sudden deterioration in vital signs or mental status
- Pneumoperitoneum
- Gross bowel distention or cecal distention over 14 cm in diameter
- Extravasation of contrast on Gastrografin enema or small bowel follow-through
- Mesenteric artery occlusion
- Intra-abdominal hemorrhage

---

**FACT BOX 52**

By the Law of Laplace (P=2T/r) wall tension is equal to pressure x radius therefore the part of the bowel with the largest diameter is subject to perforation (i.e., the cecum)

## Acute Right Lower Quadrant Pain (Appendicitis)

### History

- Abdominal pain first begins in the epigastrium, then gradually moves to the umbilicus (visceral afferents).
- The pain subsequently localizes to the RLQ (peritoneal irritation).
- Anorexia, nausea, and vomiting are common.

### Physical Exam

- After localization of the pain to the RLQ, there is tenderness to palpation and rebound.

*Guarding* occurs when there is localized peritonitis.

---

**FACT BOX 53**

**Pathophysiology of Appendicitis**

Obstruction of the appendiceal lumen (fecalith, adenopathy) leads to distention (visceral pain). This leads to lymphatic, venous, and finally arterial congestion/occlusion. Ischemia and perforation are the end results.

---

### Labs

- CBC, UA, BMP, and bHCG

### Radiology

- Acute abdominal series (usually not helpful)

### Treatment

- Hospitalize and observe.
- Laparotomy is not indicated in salpingitis, epididymitis, urinary stone, giardiasis, ruptured ovarian cyst.

*Laparotomy obligatory in:*

- Ectopic pregnancy —Salpingectomy
- Meckel's Diverticulum—Resection
- Leaking Aneurysm—Aneurysmectomy
- Impending Bowel Perforation—Colectomy
- Appendicitis—Appendectomy (if ruptured the wound is left open for drainage)

---

**FACT BOX 54**

**Ruptured Appendix**
Antibiotics are indicated and targeted for anaerobic organisms (cefotetan).

---

## Differential Diagnosis in Appendicitis

There are many pathologies that can masquerade as an acute appendicitis. The accepted false positive rate is 15%. That is, 15% of the time the patient will not have an appendicitis.

These situations may be the result of

- Mesenteric adenitis
- Crohn's disease
- Omental torsion
- Intussusception
- Lymphoma
- Diverticulitis

---

**FACT BOX 55**

If laparotomy identifies a normal appendix, look for:
- Meckel's diverticulum
- Terminal ileitis
- Mesenteric adenitis

---

## Carcinoid Tumor of Appendix

APUD cells.

Most common location is appendix.

### *Characteristics*

- <1 cm have 2% risk of metastasis.
- 1–2 cm have 50% rate of metastasis.
- >2 cm have a 90% risk of metastasis.

### *Management*

- Appendiceal carcinoids <2 cm can be treated with appendectomy.
- Carcinoids >2 cm should be treated with a right hemicolectomy.

# 23

# Acute GI Bleed

### *Statistics*

- 85% stop bleeding spontaneously.
- 25% rebleed after admission.
- 20% require surgery to stop the bleeding.
- <5% mortality with first bleed.
- 30% mortality with rebleed.

### *Anatomy*

- Upper GI from mouth to ligament of Treitz (i.e., upper GI bleeding is proximal to ligament of Treitz)
- Lower GI bleed can be from ligament of Treitz to anus

## Upper GI Bleeds

### *Etiology*

- Duodenal ulcer (30%–40%)
- Gastric ulcer (10%–20%)
- Gastritis (10%–20%)
- Esophageal varices (10%)
- Mallory-Weiss tear (10%)

### *Signs of Significant Blood Loss*

- Orthostasis
- Hypovolemic shock

- Mental statue changes
- Decreased urine output

### Resuscitation

- Two large-bore IVs (16 G–18 G)
- Crystalloid (usually 2 L LR)
- Labs (CBC, PT/pTT, T&C 4 units PRBC)
- Oxygen (may require intubation)
- Administer PRBC
- NG tube insertion

---

**FACT BOX 56**

Symptoms of UGI bleed:
- Painful bleeding suggests PUD, esophagitis, or tumor.
- Painless bleeding suggests varices, angiodysplasia.

---

**FACT BOX 57**

Symptoms of LGI bleed:
- Painful bleeding suggests colitis, hemorrhoid, anal fissure, or ischemia.
- Painless bleeding suggests diverticulosis, angiodysplasia, tumor, or hemorrhoids.

---

### History

A history of prior bleeding may suggest the cause but cannot be assumed to be the same. Medical problems including chronic renal failure, DM, COPD, peripheral vascular disease, chronic liver disease, valvular heart disease, and bleeding diathesis may be suggestive of the underlying pathology.

- Hematemesis with bright red blood or coffee-ground material suggests that the bleeding is UGI within the reach of the endoscope.

130

- Melenic stools usually arise above the ligament of Treitz but may also occur from the small intestine or ascending colon.
- Bright red blood per rectum may result from UGI or LGI bleed. If UGI bleed is associated with major hemorrhage and hemodynamic instability, if red blood appears on the toilet paper or coats the stool it suggests rectal or perianal pathology.

### Medications Associated with UGI Bleeding

- NSAIDs
- Aspirin
- Anticoagulants
- EtOH
- Methotrexate

### Physical Exam

Assess for any underlying cause of UGI bleeding.
- Mental status changes may suggest hypovolemic shock, intoxication, hepatic encephalopathy, renal failure, hyper/hypoglycemia.
- Stigmata of chronic liver disease and portal hypertension.
- Skin for petechiae and bruising.
- Abdomen for hepatosplenomegaly, surgical scars, ascites.
- Rectal exam for stool color, masses, hemoccult.

### Labs

- CBC (for H&H but may take 6 hours for Hgb to decrease, platelets will also decrease during acute bleed)
- PT/PTT (assess for underlying coagulopathy)
- T&C
- CMP (LFT [cirrhosis], bicarbonate [acidosis, ischemic bowel], BUN/Cr [renal failure], electrolytes, glucose)

### Diagnosis

- *NG Tube.* The presence of nonbloody bile-stained material excludes UGI bleed.
- *Rectal.* A black stool usually indicates a proximal bleed, maroon bloody stool indicates a bleed from the small bowel or

proximal colon. Red bloody stool usually indicates bleeding from the distal half of the large bowel.

---

FACT BOX 58

General Operative Indications
- Hemorrhage
- Obstruction
- Perforation
- Ischemia

---

### Management

- Replace clotting factors as needed
- PRBC to correct blood losses
- Antacids and $H_2$ blockers for acute gastritis
- Vasopressin drip—stops bleeding in 75% of cases (Nitro drip concurrently in patients with CAD)
- Gastric lavage should be performed when blood is obtained from the NGT to clear clot from the stomach and help stop the bleeding.

#### Diagnostic and Therapeutic Interventions

*Endoscopy.* Esophagogastroduodenoscopy (EGD) is the method of choice to evaluate UGI bleeding. This method helps to identify the cause, site, rate of bleeding and provides for therapeutic intervention. This can be done with electrocautery, or injection of the bleeding site with a sclerotic agent or epinephrine.

*Angiography.* Used for evaluation of GI bleed with normal endoscopy, suspicion of aortoenteric fistula. Alternative to surgery for high risk or patients who could not tolerate surgical intervention. Allows for identification of the bleeding with the possibility of embolization of the causative vessel.

*Surgery.* When blood loss exceeds 6 units in a 24 hour period.
- Ligation of gastroduodenal artery—duodenal ulcer disease
- Vagotomy and pyloroplasty—gastritis and PUD

- Vagotomy and antrectomy—gastritis and PUD
- Portosystemic shunt—esophageal varices

---

**FACT BOX 59**

Surgery is indicated for uncontrollable bleeding requiring >6 units of blood in 24 hours, 3–4 units if rebleed and/or rare blood type.

Mortality increases significantly if blood loss is >7 units

---

*Differential Diagnosis*

*Esophageal Varices*—Presents as painless, massive bleeding in a patient with liver disease or portal hypertension. Diagnosed with esophagogastroduodenoscopy (EGD). Treatment is sclerotherapy, vasopressin drip, balloon tamponade, portosystemic shunt (high mortality with active bleeding varices).

*Esophagitis*—Presents with heartburn, chest pain, dysphagia, odynophagia, hoarseness, aspiration. Etiology includes reduced LES tone, delayed gastric emptying, infection (herpes, CMV, candidia) toxins (EtOH, caustic agents, potassium tablets). Diagnose with barium swallow to identify hiatus hernia or esophagitis, EGD, esophageal manometry, acid perfusion test, esophageal pH monitor. Treatment is limited to $H_2$ blockers and antacids. Acute bleeding resolves on its own in 85% of cases.

*Mallory-Weiss Tear*—A longitudinal mucosal tear at the esophagogastric junction. Presents with history of vomiting or retching. EtOH frequently associated. Diagnose with EGD showing a linear tear with active bleeding. Treatment is coagulation with electrocautery, intra-arterial vasopressin; however, the majority will stop bleeding within 24–48 hours.

*Gastritis*—Erosion of mucosa by irritants: acid, bile, medications, toxins. Patients present with painless bleeding, history of aspirin or irritant ingestion. Diagnose with EGD and treat with $H_2$ blockers and antacids to keep pH >4. Selective arterial vasopressin. Gastrectomy may be required in cases of uncontrollable exsanguinating hemorrhage.

> **FACT BOX 60**
>
> Prophylaxis of gastritis or PUD with
> - Famotidine (Pepcid) 20 mg IV q12h
> - Ranitidine (Zantac) 50 mg IV q6–8h (drip 6.25 mg/h)
> - Sucralfate (Carafate) 1 g PO q6h
> - Mylanta 15 mL q4h for pH <4

*Acutely Bleeding Peptic Ulcer*—Presents with history of PUD, nausea, crampy abdominal pain, diarrhea. Diagnose with EGD. Treat with $H_2$ blockers, endoscopic hemostasis (electrode, heater probe, laser), intra-arterial vasopressin, or embolization.

*Gastric Angiodysplasia*—Presents with painless bleeding. Patient may have a history of renal disease or hereditary telangiectasia. Diagnose with EGD. Treat with coagulation via heater probe, electrode, YAG laser.

*Aortoenteric Fistula*—Presents usually with massive painless bleeding but may be chronic and intermittent. Patients with abdominal aortic aneurysm (AAA) or history of repair of AAA (results from pressure and erosion at the vascular anastomosis into an adjacent segment of bowel). Diagnose with upper endoscopy (to rule out other causes of bleeding), angiography, surgical exploration in cases of suspected aortoenteric fistula where other causes of bleeding are not found. Treatment is the replacement of the vascular segment and repair of the fistula.

**Lower GI Bleeds**

*Etiology*

- Diverticulosis
- Angiodysplasia
- Cancer

> **FACT BOX 61**
>
> Most common cause of LGI bleed is a UGI bleed.

## Labs

• CBC, PT/pTT, T&C, CHEM 18

## Diagnosis

• Place NG tube—rule out UGI source of blood loss.
• Rectal exam.
• Anoscopy.

## Diagnostic and Therapeutic Interventions

*Sigmoidoscopy*—Rigid is better, should be a part of the initial exam. Distinguishes perirectal bleeding (hemorrhoids, colitis, rectal cancer ) from a more proximal site of bleeding.

*Colonoscopy*—Difficult during active bleeding and usually accomplished days after bleeding stopped.

*Angiography*—Detects bleeds at a rate of 1–2 mL/min. It is helpful to perform a nuclear bleeding scan prior because if it is normal the yield of angiography is low. Important whenever surgery is considered because it will direct the surgeon's attention to either the right or left colon.

*Therapeutic Angiography*—Vasopressin and embolization are important modalities for controlling bleeding.

*Tagged RBC Scan*—This can detect bleeding at a rate of 0.1–0.5 mL/min or greater.

*Surgery*—Hemicolectomy is considered in cases of life-threatening hemorrhage that cannot be controlled by other means.

## Differential Diagnosis

*UGI Source*—The number one cause of lower GI bleed is an upper GI bleed. Always insert an NG tube to evaluate for an UGI source.

*Hemorrhoids*—Diagnose external hemorrhoids by direct visualization where internal require anoscope to visualize. Diagnosis of hemorrhoidal bleeding can only be established if active bleeding is observed or there is fresh clot overlying the hemorrhoid. In all other cases a more thorough examination of the colon must be undertaken. Treatment is injection of sclerosing agent, banding, hemorrhoidectomy, stool softeners.

*Diverticulosis*—Extrusion of the mucosa through the muscular layer of the intestinal wall at the site of penetrating blood vessels. Most occur in the sigmoid, but may occur anywhere. Most bleeding comes from diverticula of the right colon. Presentation is with passage of stool with bright red or maroon clots. Usually painless. In patients who have stopped bleeding BE can show the diverticula. In cases of massive bleeding colonoscopy may be difficult to visualize and tagged RBC scan or angiography should be used. Bleeding usually stops spontaneously. Other options include intra-arterial vasopressin, heater probe, or electrocautery. Surgery is indicated if persistent bleeding cannot be controlled medically.

*Angiodysplasia*—A-V malformations seen as tortuous submucosal vessels. Age >50. Associated with valvular heart disease (calcific aortic stenosis) in 50% of patients. Most common in the cecum or ascending colon. Presentation of painless bright red or maroon bleeding. Diagnosis with colonoscopy, mesenteric angiography. Treatment is intra-arterial vasopressin, heater probe, electrocautery. Surgery for uncontrolled bleeding.

*Ischemic Colitis*—Causes include decreased cardiac output, shock, interruption of blood supply during surgery, thrombosis of SMA, IMA, mesenteric vein, or occasionally embolization (most common to SMA). Presents with sudden onset of abdominal pain and bleeding. Patients have history of hypotension, arrhythmia, recent MI, aortic surgery. Diagnosis via flex sigmoidoscopy (usually affects the left colon) angiography. Treatment by identification and correction of contributing factors, bowel rest, and NG suction, if bleeding stops spontaneously or colonoscopy can establish the diagnosis. Uncontrolled bleeding requires angiography for diagnostic as well as therapeutic purposes. Surgery is indicated to remove necrotic bowel.

*Neoplasia*—Presents with minor, chronic, episodic bleeding producing red or maroon stools, usually painless. Management is colonoscopy and resection.

*Meckel's Diverticulum*—Usually presents before the age of 2 years. Bleeding is painless and presents as maroon stool. Bleeding is the result of peptic ulceration of ileal mucosa (due to gastric and pancreatic tissue present). Diagnosis with scan using radiolabeled technetium, which is taken up by the gastric mucosa. Mesenteric angiography. Treatment is resection of the diverticulum.

# 24

# Peptic Ulcer Disease

**Anatomy**

Type I—lesser curvature
Type II—body of stomach and duodenum
Type III—prepyloric ulcer
Type IV—near the GE junction

## Gastric Ulcer

### History

- More common in men, the elderly, and patients of lower socioeconomic class.
- Burning epigastric pain that is relieved with food, but pain recurs 0.5 to 1.5 hours later.

### Etiology

- EtOH
- Aspirin
- NSAIDs
- Smoking
- Reflux of bile into the stomach

People with gastric ulcers have lower than normal rates of acid secretion but serum gastrin levels are elevated as much as two times normal.

## Labs

- CBC
- Serum gastrin

## Radiographic Evaluation

- UGI is the initial test and detects about 70%–80% of gastric ulcers.

## Endoscopy

- EGD can be the first line diagnostic modality in most instances. Multiple biopsies are performed to identify possible cancer (10% of gastric ulcers are malignant, but benign ulcers do *not* degenerate into cancer ). Gastric washings are also done for cytology. Endoscopy has a 95% sensitivity.

## Medical Treatment

- Most gastric ulcers will heal in 12–15 weeks.
- $H_2$ blockers are effective especially in patients with normal acid secretion.
- Sulcrafate (Carafate) under acidic conditions binds to the damaged mucosa and is effective in gastric ulcer treatment.
- Patients should avoid EtOH, tobacco, and irritating drugs.
- A recurrence rate of 25%–60% in 5 years is associated with short-term medical treatment. Recurrences are within 6 months.

## Surgical Treatment

Indications are:
- Malignancy
- Perforation
- Hemorrhage
- Obstruction
- Refractory to medical therapy
- Recurrence

## *Surgical Procedures*

- Hemigastrectomy—Resection of the distal 50%–60% of the stomach with excision of the ulcer, with gastroduodenostomy (Billroth I) reconstruction. A gastrojejunostomy (Billroth II) is done if the duodenum cannot be mobilized enough to create a tension-free anastomosis. 1%–10% mortality and 5%–10% recurrence
- Truncal Vagotomy with Antrectomy—Both are acid-reducing procedures and eliminate parasympathetic innervation to the stomach and remove the gastrin-producing cell of the antrum resulting in decreased acid secretion. 1%–10% mortality and 1% recurrence

## Duodenal Ulcer

### *History*

- Tobacco, caffeine, EtOH, and aspirin.
- Blood type O and nonsecreters are at higher risk.

### *Etiology*

- The major cause is increased acid production.
- Parietal cells are more sensitive to gastrin and secrete more acid.
- *Helicobacter pylori.*

### *Symptoms*

- History of epigastric pain that radiates to the back and is relieved by food. The pain typically wakes the patient up at night.

> **FACT BOX 62**
>
> Duodenal ulcers are rarely malignant.

## *Radiographic Evaluation*

- UGI

## Endoscopy

- EGD can provide accurate diagnosis of duodenal ulcers and therapeutic intervention if bleeding is present.

## Treatment

- Avoidance of the offending agents tobacco, EtOH, caffeine, and aspirin is recommended.
- Antacids and $H_2$ blockers (since recurrence is common following discontinuation, maintenance therapy is recommended).
- *Helicobacter pylori* treatment.

## Surgical Treatment

Indications are:
- Refractory to medical management
- Complications (perforation, hemorrhage, obstruction)

## Operative Procedures

- Truncal Vagotomy with Antrectomy—1%–10% mortality and 1% recurrence
- Truncal Vagotomy with Pyloroplasty—Vagotomy decreases acid secretion, but also decreases motility that is overcome by pyloroplasty. 1%–7% mortality and 7%–10% recurrence
- Selective Vagotomy—Decreases acid secretion while leaving motility intact. 0.1%–1% mortality and 10% recurrence

| TABLE 24.1 Anti-Ulcer Surgery: Morbidity/Mortality | |
|---|---|
| **In order of operative morbidity/mortality (lowest to highest)** | **In order of recurrence (lowest to highest)** |
| Selective vagotomy | Vagotomy/antrectomy |
| Vagotomy/pyloroplasty | Vagotomy/pyloroplasty |
| Vagotomy/antrectomy | Selective vagotomy |

### Long-Term Complications of Surgery for Peptic Ulcer Disease

*Dumping Syndrome*—Occurs with all procedures except selective vagotomy. The initiating event is rapid gastric emptying and symptoms of nausea/vomiting/diarrhea, dyspepsia, epigastric pain, flushing, tachycardia, dizziness, diaphoresis. This is thought to be due to duodenal/jejunal distention from the food bolus, volume contraction from fluid displacement onto the hyperosmolar solution in the gut, and the release of vaso-active hormones (serotonin, bradykinin, VIP). Usual treatment is dietary. Symptoms are transient in most cases.

*Postvagotomy Diarrhea*—This is very common. Treatment is dietary/medical after other causes of diarrhea have been ruled out.

*Weight Loss*—The causes are usually early satiety after gastrectomy. Also diarrhea and blind loop syndrome can result after Billroth II from bacterial overgrowth and malabsorption of fats, calcium, and vitamins D and B-12. Treatment is with po metronidazole or conversion to Billroth I.

*Anemia*—Lack of iron from malabsorption following gastric resection or persistent ulceration and bleeding. B-12 deficiency from atrophic gastritis or blind loop syndrome. Folate deficiency is uncommon but can be caused by malabsorption.

*Alkaline Reflux Gastritis/Esophagitis*—This is caused by reflux of bile into the gastric remnant. It can be treated with cholestyramine or Roux-en-Y jejunal interposition.

*Afferent Loop Syndrome*—This occurs after Billroth II. Pancreatic and biliary secretions collect in a partially obstructed afferent loop causing distention and pain followed by projectile vomiting. Management requires surgical revision of the gastrojejunal anastomosis.

### Complications of Ulcers

*Perforation* usually occurs with ulcers on the anterior duodenum. Closure of the defect with a patch of omentum (Graham patch) and definitive treatment with vagotomy/antrectomy is the usual course of action if there is minimal soilage of the peritoneal cavity.

*Hemorrhage* can result and can usually be controlled by medical management. EGD is necessary to evaluate the site of the bleed. Electrocautery through the scope may be able to stop the bleeding. Surgery is required to stop massive hemorrhage (>1500 cc of blood products required or >6 units of blood needed over a 24-hour period). Studies have indicated that mortality increases significantly as the number of units transfused in a 24-hour period rises. Surgery in these cases involves oversewing the bleeding point or if necessary ligating the gastroduodenal artery. Definitive procedures are also done at this point including vagotomy/pyloroplasty.

*Gastric outlet obstruction* is treated with several days of NG suction followed by vagotomy/antrectomy or vagotomy/pyloroplasty.

# 25

# Inflammatory Bowel Disease

## Types of Inflammatory Bowel Diseases

There are two divisions of inflammatory bowel diseases (IBD):
Crohn's disease
Ulcerative colitis

**TABLE 25.1**
**Characteristics of Inflammatory Bowel Disease**

| Characteristics | Crohn's Disease | Ulcerative Colitis |
| --- | --- | --- |
| Location | Entire GI tract | Rectum; then colon |
| Pattern | Transmural, segmental | Isolated to the mucosa |
| Bleeding | Rare | Common |
| Complications | Fistula, stricture | Toxic megacolon |
| Carcinoma | Some increased risk with long-term disease | Increased incidence |

## Ulcerative Colitis

Mucosal inflammation with almost invariable rectal involvement. The inflammation is continuous without anal or perianal disease. Pseudopolyps and/or crypt abscess can be seen on histology.

---

FACT BOX 63

The risk of colon cancer increases by 2% at 10 years of disease and increases by 2% each year thereafter.

---

## History

Extraintestinal manifestations include:
- Arthritis
- Aphthous stomatitis
- Sclerosing cholangitis
- Iritis and episcleritis
- Ankylosing spondylitis and sacroileitis

## Symptoms

### General

- Bloody diarrhea
- Cramping and abdominal pain
- Malaise, fever, weight loss, and anemia

### Toxic Megacolon

- Dilatation of transverse colon
- Abdominal pain, tender with distention
- Fever, leukocytosis, hypoalbuminemia
- Significant risk of perforation

## Lab

- CBC
- Stool samples for enteric pathogens (ova, parasites, *C. difficile* toxin, etc.)

## Radiology

- Abdominal Radiology—To assess possible colonic dilatation
- Small bowel contrast studies to identify possible Crohn's disease with involvement of small bowel

### Endoscopy

- Proctoscopy—Mucosal inflammation at the dentate line. Avoid colonoscopy and or barium enema if fulminate colitis suspected due to increased risk of perforation.

### Treatment

- Steroids
- Sulfasalazine 500 mg PO qid
- Mesalamine (5 ASA) 800 mg PO tid
- 6-mercaptopurine

### Indications for Surgery

- Hemorrhage
- Perforation
- Toxic megacolon refractory to intensive medical management
- Dysplasia or cancer

### Procedures

*Total Proctocolectomy with Permanent End Ileostomy*—Removes the rectum and colon

*Total Proctocolectomy with J Pouch and Ileoanal Anastomosis*—Currently the most common procedure for UC. Temporary loop ileostomy for 10 weeks while anal anastomosis heals. Requires a second operation to take the ileostomy down.

*Abdominal Colectomy with Hartmann's Pouch*—Total colectomy with closure of the rectum making a blind pouch.

*Total Proctocolectomy and Continent (Kock) Ileostomy*—Ileal reservoir with a valve is created.

Patient will be required to intubate the ileostomy 4–6 times throughout the day to remove stool. In procedures that leave the rectum, patients will need to have regular proctoscopy to survey for recurrence of UC or cancer.

**Crohn's Colitis**

Transmural inflammation that is segmental in nature with skip lesions. The ileocecal junction is the most common site but can be anywhere in the GI tract.

- Up to 35% will experience perianal disease including fistula and abscess formation.
- Granulomas present in 30%–50%.
- Linear ulcers may coalesce with transverse fissures giving the characteristic cobblestone appearance.
- Risk of colon cancer is less than than of UC.

---

**FACT BOX 64**

An accurate diagnosis of UC is essential as total proctocolectomy *is* curative in UC; however, it is not in Crohn's and may cause significant morbidity.

---

### *Extraintestinal Characteristics*

- Arthritis
- Aphthous stomatitis
- Sclerosing cholangitis
- Iritis and episcleritis
- Ankylosing spondylitis and sacroileitis

### *History*

- Fistulas between bowel and bladder (enterovesical fistula), vagina (enterovaginal fistula), skin (enterocutaneous fistula), or other intestinal segments (enteroenteric fistula)
- Anal abscess and fistulas
- Abdominal abscess (often in the RLQ)
- Fulminate colitis

### *Symptoms*

- Diarrhea
- Crampy abdominal pain
- Malaise, fever, leukocytosis, weight loss

## Labs

- Stool Samples—Identify ova, parasites, or infectious etiology.

## Radiology

- Barium Enema — Establish extent of disease.
- Small Bowel Follow-through—To identify possible Crohn's disease with involvement of small bowel.

## Endoscopy

- Proctoscopy—If the rectal tissue is not involved UC can virtually be eliminated as diagnosis.
- Colonoscopy—Helpful to establish the extent of colonic involvement.

## Medical Treatment

- Steroids.
- Immunosuppressive agents (6-MP, azathioprine).
- Metronidazole (Flagyl) 500 mg IV/PO tid (unknown mechanism).
- TPN—Bowel rest induces remission in some patients with significant Crohn's.

## Surgical Indications

- Obstruction
- Anorectal abscess or fistula
- Fulminate colitis
- Hemorrhage
- Cancer (less likely than with UC)

## Surgical Procedure

- Take narrow margins to preserve bowel. Only grossly involved bowel should be resected.
- Ileoanal anastomosis with J pouch is contraindicated secondary to the high incidence of pouchitis (infection and inflammation of the ileal pouch).

- 50% recur in 5 years after resection at the site of anastomosis (i.e., resection is *not* curative, only palliative).
- Partially stenosed areas of small bowel may be opened up using stricturoplasty to avoid further bowel resection.

# 26

# Esophagus

**Esophageal Cancer**

*Statistics*

- 90% are squamous cell cancer (upper half).
- 5% are adenocarcinoma (originates from Barrett's esophagus in lower half).
- 20% potentially curable at presentation.

*History*

The typical patient is a 55-year-old black male with 30 pack a year smoking history who reports "occasional EtOH" and now complains of dysphagia for liquids and solids increasing over the past 3 months.
- Black
- Male
- Smoker
- EtOH
- Radiation
- Caustic ingestion
- Barrett's
- Plummer-Vinson

*Signs and Symptoms*

- Dysphagia (difficulty with swallowing) initially to solids and progressing to liquids

- Odynophagia (painful swallowing)
- Back pain
- Weight loss
- Aspiration
- Recurrent pneumonia

### Radiologic Evaluation

- Barium swallow shows an asymmetric narrowing.

### Endoscopy

- EGD with cytology and biopsy to make a histological diagnosis

### Staging

- Bronchoscopy to evaluate for tracheal invasion
- CT scan of chest and abdomen

### Unresectable Tumors

- Horner's syndrome
- Phrenic nerve paralysis
- Hoarseness (recurrent laryngeal nerve damage)
- Malignant pleural effusion
- Tracheal invasion
- Distant mets (stage IV)

### Treatment

Surgery (esophagectomy), radiotherapy (XRT), and chemotherapy

#### Surgical Procedures

*Ivor-Lewis*—Done via midline abdominal incision and right thoracotomy. The stomach is mobilized and brought into the thorax. A gastroesophageal anastomosis is made in the chest or neck.

*Transhiatal*—Accomplished via abdominal and neck incisions. Blunt esophagectomy, gastric mobilization, and reanastomosis in the neck.

*Interposition graft*—Reconstruction of the esophagus can also be accomplished with bowel interposition (jejunal or colonic) graft.

*Palliation* with stent, laser ablation, surgery, or XRT.

### Prognosis

- 80% mortality at 1 year
- <10% 5-year survival

## Esophagus

### Anatomy

- C6-T11
- 24 cm in length (~40 cm from the incisors to the LES)

### Arterial Supply

- Inferior thyroid
- Bronchial, intercostal
- Inferior phrenic
- Left gastric

### Lower Esophageal Sphincter

**TABLE 26.1**
**Lower Esophageal Sphincter Control**

| Increased Tone | Decreased Tone |
| --- | --- |
| Protein | Fat, chocolate |
| High pH | Low pH |
| Vasopressin | Secretin |
| Cholinergics | NTG |
| Gastrin | Glucagon |

## Gastroesophageal Reflux Disease (GERD)

Secondary to dysfunction of the LES resulting in recurrent reflux into the distal esophagus.

## *Etiologies*

- Decreased LES tone
- Hiatal hernia
- Scleroderma
- Pregnancy

## *Symptoms*

- Substernal pain
- Heartburn that worsens with bending over or the supine position

## *Diagnosis*

- EGD
- Esophageal manometry
- 24-hour pH monitoring

## *Treatment: Medical*

- Antacids
- $H_2$ blockers
- Eliminate smoking, alcohol
- Elevation of head of bed
- No food 3 hours before bedtime

## *Indications for Surgery*

- Refractory to medical management
- Esophagitis
- Barrett's esophagus
- Stricture

## *Surgical Antireflux Procedures*

*Laparoscopic Nissen Fundoplication*—Currently the standard first line surgical technique if no contraindications to laparoscopic surgery. 360-degree wrap of the fundus around the distal esophagus. Provides the advantage of decreased hospital stay, recovery time, and morbidity with equivalent results compared to open procedures.

*Nissen Fundoplication*—360-degree wrap of fundus around esophagus performed through abdominal incision.

*Belsey Mark IV*—270-degree wrap performed through a left thoracotomy.

*Hill Repair* (posterior gastroplexy)—Uses arcuate ligament to re-establish the intra-abdominal position of the LES.

## Other Esophageal Disorders

### Cricopharyngeal Dysfunction

Failure of the upper esophageal sphincter (cricopharyngeous muscle) to relax properly. May result in a pharyngoesophageal (Zenker's) diverticulum. Often associated with hiatal hernia and GER.

*Treatment*

- Cricopharyngeal myotomy

### Achalasia

Dysfunction of LES resulting in a failure of relaxation. CA of the esophagus is $10\times$ more common in patients with achalasia.

*Treatment*

- *Pneumatic Dilatation*—temporizing in that repeated dilatations are required. Risk of perforation or rupture.
- *Esophagomyotomy (modified Heller procedure)*—Can be done either open or laparoscopically

### Caustic Ingestions

Typically result from ingestion of chemical (alkali or acid). Ingestion of alkali is worse because there is no buffer in stomach. Acid can be partially buffered by stomach contents. Long-term complication of stricture formation. Patients should be evaluated with EGD or barium swallow early after ingestion.

*Treatment*

- Steroids and antibiotics for 3 weeks
- Repeated dilatation of stricture

### Boerhaave's Syndrome

Represents a longitudinal full-thickness esophageal rupture. Presents with crepitation, crunching heart sounds (Hamman's sign), septic shock. Patient complains of chest pain, dysphagia, nausea, fever, tachycardia.

*Labs*

- Elevated amylase

*Diagnosis*

- CXR
- Gastrografin swallow

---

**FACT BOX 65**

Rupture is most common on the left.

---

*Treatment*

- Surgical repair and drainage
- Antibiotics

### Esophageal Webs

- Plummer-Vinson syndrome upper esophageal webs (female, edentulous, atrophic oral mucosa, anemia, dysphagia)
- Schatzki's rings lower esophageal webs

### Hiatal Hernia

*Type I (Sliding)*

- Most common type
- Reflux symptoms

*Type II (Paraesophageal)*

- Gastric fundus herniating alongside the esophagus.
- May cause incarceration or strangulation.
- All of these should be repaired.

# 27

# Gastric Cancer

**Risks**

- Achlorhydria (partial gastrectomy, atrophic gastritis, pernicious anemia)
- Gastric polyps
- Smoked foods

**Signs and Symptoms**

- Early satiety
- Gastric outlet obstruction (vomiting)
- Ulcers
- Weight loss
- Anemia

**Signs**

- Supraclavicular node (Virchow's node)
- Umbilical node (Sister Mary Joseph's node)

**Workup**

- UGI reveals gastric mass or ulcer.
- EGD with biopsy and cytology.
- CT for extent of spread.

## Pathology

*Adenocarcinoma* (78%)
- Ulcerating (most common)
- Fungating (least common)
- Linitis plastica (worst prognosis)
- Superficial spreading

*Gastric lymphoma* (10%)

*Leiomyosarcoma* (3%)

## Management

- Subtotal or total gastrectomy for cure. Surgery for palliation of gastric outlet obstruction
- Chemotherapy (FAM-5-FU, Adriamycin, MMC) for palliation

## Prognosis

- 40% eligible for curative surgery at presentation
- <5% 5-year overall survival

# 28

# Colon Cancer

## Statistics

- Second leading cause of cancer deaths.
- 10% of all colorectal cancers can be found by digital rectal exam.
- 3%–6% of patients will have a synchronous lesion in the colon.
- 90% of all colorectal cancers are sporadic, 10% genetic or familial.
- 5% risk in the United States of developing colorectal cancer.

## Genetics (see Molecular Surgery)

Hereditary nonpolyposis colorectal carcinoma (HNPCC)
- Lynch I—autosomal dominant
- Lynch II—associated with ovary, breast, stomach cancers

## Genes

It is suggested that colorectal cancer develops from a progression from benign adenomas who develop genetic mutations or loss of heterozygosity (LOC)
- *ras* gene mutation (oncogene)
- Chromosome 5q—APC
- Chromosome 17p—p53 (tumor suppressor gene)

- Chromosome 18q—DCC (deleted in colorectal carcinoma)
- Chromosome 2p—hMSH2
- Chromosome 3—hMSH1

## Risks

- High-fat diet
- Low fiber
- Older age
- Family history
- Ulcerative colitis (patients at 10 years have 1%–2% chance of cancer per year)

---

**FACT BOX 66**

Right-sided lesions present with anemia.
Left-sided lesions present with changes in stool caliber or obstruction.

---

## Signs and Symptoms

- Iron deficiency anemia
- LGI bleeding
- Hemoccult positive
- Constipation
- Diarrhea alternating with constipation
- Pencil-thin stools
- Tenesmus
- Bowel obstruction
- Perforation

## Diagnostic Studies

---

**FACT BOX 67**

Digital rectal exam can identify as many as 6% of all colorectal cancers.

---

**Labs**

- CBC
- LFT
- Calcium
- CEA (baseline)

---

FACT BOX **68**

Occult blood on DRE is associated with colon cancer in 10% of patients.

---

**Radiology**

- Barium enema
- Sigmoidoscopy with biopsy
- Colonoscopy with biopsy

**Colon Polyps**

- Tubular (5% malignant)
- Tubulovillous (25% malignant)
- Villous (50% malignant)

---

FACT BOX **69**

Rectal bleeding in patients >30 years old is rectal cancer until proven otherwise.

---

**Size and Risk of Malignancy**

- 1% of polyps <1 cm are malignant.
- 50% of polyps >2 cm are malignant.

**Staging Workup**

- Physical exam to assess for bone pain (bone scan if positive), mental status changes (CT of head)
- CXR
- LFT (CT of abdomen and pelvis if abnormal)

TABLE 28.1
Colorectal Cancer Staging—Duke's Classification

| Stage | Description |
| --- | --- |
| A | Confined to the mucosa |
| B1 | Into but not through the muscularis propria |
| B2 | Through the muscularis propria |
| C1 | Into but not through the muscularis propria with positive nodes |
| C2 | Through the muscularis propria with positive nodes |
| D | Metastasis |

**Treatment**

Surgical resection for:
- Polyps found to be sessile and invasive
- Polyp with stalk involvement
- Poor histology
- Resection of involved bowel with 2-cm margins along with the lymphovascular pedicle
- Adjuvant chemotherapy and/or radiation

**Procedures**

Cecum and ascending colon
- *Right hemicolectomy.* Resect distal ileum to mid-transverse colon with ileocolic, right and middle colic with mesentery

Left transverse colon to splenic flexure
- *Extended right hemicolectomy* or *transverse colectomy.* Resect transverse and proximal descending colon with middle and left colic arteries

Descending and sigmoid colon
- *Left hemicolectomy* or *sigmoid colectomy.* Resect from splenic flexure to rectosigmoid with left colic and sigmoidal arteries

Proximal third of rectum
- *Anterior resection*

5–10 cm from anal verge
- *Low anterior resection or abdominal-sacral resection*

Distal third of rectum
- *Abdominoperineal resection* (Miles procedure) with sigmoid colostomy. Low anterior resection with re-anastomosis if >4 cm of rectal tissue remains.

**Follow-Up**

- CEA every 2 months for 2 years, then every 4 months for 2 years, then annually.
- Colonoscopy within the first 2–3 months, then annually.
- LFTs every 3 months for 2 years, then every 6 months for 2 years, then annually.
- CXR every 6 months for 3 years, then annually.

# 29

# Anorectal Disorders

**Anal Fissure**

*Symptoms*

- Anal pain associated with defecation with or without bleeding

*Diagnosis*

- Digital rectal exam
- Anoscopy to inspect the anal canal
- Fissure at posterior midline

---

FACT BOX **70**

Atypical lateral location could be Crohn's disease.

---

*Treatment*

- Fiber products to produce soft bowel movement (Citrucel, Metamucil)
- Xylocaine 2% gel plus hot Sitz baths for pain relief.
- Surgery for closed lateral sphincterotomy.

**External Hemorrhoids**

These are not really hemorrhoids but actually all are perianal skin tags. Most often they become symptomatic when a small perianal blood vessel ruptures on straining and results in perianal hematoma.

### Symptoms

- Bluish tender mass externally in perianal area next to anus
- Constant pain with sudden onset

### Treatment

- Excision under local anesthesia. Excise small ellipse of skin so hematoma does not re-accumulate. Do not close incision (pack).

## Internal Hemorrhoids

### Etiology

- Engorgement of anal cushions
- Prolonged straining during defecation and increased abdominal pressure

### Symptoms

- Rectal bleeding
- Prolapse
- With or without itching

### Diagnosis

- Digital rectal exam.
- Proctoscopy (anoscopy).
- Must exclude higher pathology by barium enema or colonoscopy. Always consider neoplastic process with rectal bleeding until ruled out.

---

**FACT BOX 71**

Locations of hemorrhoids
- Right anterolateral
- Right posterolateral
- Left lateral

---

## *Assess Prolapse*

- First degree—bleed but no prolapse.
- Second degree—bleed and prolapse but spontaneously reduce
- Third degree—bleed and prolapse and must be manually reduced
- Fourth degree—prolapsed and cannot be reduced manually

## *Treatment*

- Increased fiber and stool softeners
- Rubber band ligation
- Sclerotherapy
- Photocoagulation
- Hemorrhoidectomy

## Pilonidal Disease

### *Symptoms*

- Pain
- Erythema
- Purulent drainage above gluteal crease

### *Diagnosis*

- Examine for pilonidal pits
- Proctoscopy to exclude fistula in ano

### *Treatment*

- Drainage under local anesthesia or antibiotics (often unsuccessful).
- Definitive treatment is surgical excision.
- Anal fistulae that extend posteriorly may be fistula in ano. Examine the canal.

## Fistula

### *Etiology*

- Fistulae are cryptoglandular in origin, beginning in the anal glands and emptying into the anal crypts.

- Located between the anal crypt and perianal skin.
- Most common site of internal opening is posterior anal crypt.

*Goodsall's Rule*

- External openings posterior to a transverse line bisecting the anus connect to the posterior midline crypt by a curvilinear line. External openings anterior to this line will communicate to an anterior crypt by a short direct tract.

### Symptoms

- Purulent drainage from perianal area
- Abscess

### Physical Exam

- Proctoscopy and rectal exam of anal canal. Most internal fistula openings are hard to find but can usually be felt as a small hard area in the anal canal (finger to DIP joint).

### Treatment

- Surgery is fistulotomy with laying open of fistula tract.
- If large amount of sphincter is involved, delayed sphincterotomy with Seton insertion is necessary.
- Fistulotomy may result in permanent incontinence if not carefully done.
- If multiple fistulae present consider Crohn's disease or hidradenitis suppurativa.

## Abscess

### Anatomy

- Most abscesses originate from fistulae and are intersphincteric.
- Inferior extension results in perianal abscess.
- Lateral extension results in ischiorectal fossa abscess.
- Superior extension results in supralevator abscess.

## Etiology

- Most abscesses arise from fistulae in ano.
- The internal opening has already closed in most patients at the time of abscess drainage.
- If patient gets recurrent abscess at the same site weeks to months later, a fistula is always present and the patient should have definitive fistulotomy.

## Symptoms

- Painful
- Erythematous
- Swelling in perianal area
- With or without fever

## Diagnosis

- Physical exam
- Aspirate with large bore needle if necessary

## Treatment

- Drain under local anesthesia.
- If too painful for patient, a large abscess, or a diabetic or immunocompromised patient, take him or her to the OR for surgical drainage.

# 30

# Liver

## Anatomy

Liver is divided into 8 segments based on blood supply (portal venous system).

The interlobar fissure is an invisible line that connects the gall-bladder fossa anteriorly and the IVC posteriorly.

The falciform ligament marks the division between the median and lateral segments of the left lobe. Divides 2&3 from segment 4.

## Arterial Supply

- Celiac—common hepatic—proper hepatic—left and right hepatic
- Porta hepatis contains common bile duct and common hepatic artery (medial to lateral) with the portal vein posterior
- Hepatic artery provides 25% of blood flow
- Portal vein provides 75% of blood flow

---

**FACT BOX 72**

Triangle of Calot
- Cystic duct
- Common hepatic duct
- Lower edge of the liver

---

## Liver Function Tests

- *Synthetic function* is assessed by serum proteins albumin, prealbumin, transferrin.
- *Clotting factors* assessed by the PT/PTT.
- *Clearance* is assessed by the levels of ammonia and indirect bilirubin.
- *Patency of the biliary tree* is assessed by the levels of direct bilirubin and alkaline phosphatase.
- *Liver injury* is assessed by AST and ALT.

## Portal Hypertension

### Statistics

- 85% is caused by cirrhosis secondary to alcohol.
- 50% of UGI bleeds in cirrhotic patients are due to variceal bleeding.
- 15% of alcoholics develop cirrhosis and 30% die within a year of diagnosis.
- 40% of cirrhotic patients develop bleeding varices.

### Etiology

Portal hypertension is the elevation of portal venous pressure >6 mm Hg and is produces a variety of systemic problems. Most notably are varices that result when portal pressure exceeds 20 mm Hg and are subject to rupture and subsequent hemorrhage. Areas of variceal development include:
- Gastroesophageal junction
- Periumbilical caput medusa
- Hemorrhoids

## Cirrhosis

Cirrhosis causes 85% of portal hypertension with the most common cause related to alcohol ingestion. Metabolic sources such as Wilson's, hemochromatosis, and alpha 1 antitrypsin deficiency are uncommon causes. Schistosomiasis is the most common cause worldwide.

Other sources:
- Portal vein obstruction.
- Budd-Chiari syndrome is a hepatic vein thrombosis secondary to hypercoagulable state, OCP use, trauma.
- Constrictive pericarditis causes an increase in the IVC pressure and resistance to hepatic outflow.
- Splenic vein thrombosis is usually the result of pancreatitis or a pancreatic tumor.
- Right heart failure.

### Symptoms

- Encephalopathy
- GI hemorrhage
- Malnutrition
- Ascites
- Venous collaterals
- Splenomegaly

The most significant adverse effect of increased portosystemic circulation is the risk of variceal bleeding. Patients who have one bleed with subsequent rebleed have a mortality as high as 33%.

### Assessment

The Child's classification is used to determine operative risk for shunting procedures.

**TABLE 30.1**
**Child's Classification**

| Child's Classification | A | B | C |
| --- | --- | --- | --- |
| Serum bilirubin | <2 | 2–3 | >3 |
| Serum albumin | >3.5 | 3–3.5 | <3 |
| Ascites | Absent | Controlled | Refractory |
| Encephalopathy | Absent | Minimal | Severe |
| Malnutrition | Absent | Mild | Severe |
| Operative mortality | 2% | 10% | 50% |

### Acute Bleeding Management from Varices

- *Sclerotherapy* controls bleeding in 80% of patients with mortality of <3%.
- *Vasopressin/nitroglycerin* decreases mesenteric blood flow and nitro protects coronary circulation. Contraindicated in patients with history of ischemic heart disease.
- *Balloon tamponade* done with Sengstaken-Blakemore tube controls bleeding in 80% with rebleeding in 20% of patients when balloon is deflated. Complications include aspiration pneumonia, ischemia, and necrosis of distal esophagus. Can be minimized with periodic deflation.
- *Transjugular intrahepatic portosystemic shunt (TIPS)* created between hepatic veins and portal vein via stent placement. 10%–20% incidence of encephalopathy.

### Elective Management

Useful in patients who are not actively bleeding with the goal of surgery to prevent rebleeding.
- *TIPS*
- *Endoscopic variceal sclerosis*

### Shunting Procedures

*Nonselective Shunts*

- *End-to-side portosystemic shunt*—this is the most common operation performed. The hepatic end of the portal vein is ligated with the inferior end anastomosed to the IVC.
- *Mesocaval shunt*—a prosthetic graft connects the SMV to the IVC. Portal blood flow to the liver becomes unpredictable and blood may even flow retrograde leading to hepatic failure.
- *Side-to-side portocaval shunt*—connects the portal vein to the IVC while maintaining patency of the portal vein and flow to the liver. More difficult to perform as longer lengths of vessel must be exposed.

*Selective Portosystemic Shunts*

*Distal splenorenal shunt (Warren).* The distal end of the splenic vein is anastomosed to the left renal vein with the proximal splenic vein ligated. The following veins are ligated:
- Coronary vein
- Right gastroepiploic vein
- Proximal splenic vein

## Liver Tumors

### *Statistics*

- 50% of cancers outside the abdomen metastasize to the liver
- 10% of patients have resectable tumors at diagnosis
- 25% 5-year survival
- Most common tumor of the liver is metastatic

### *Benign Neoplasms*

*Hemangioma*

- Most common benign liver tumor.
- Usually asymptomatic but may present with RUQ pain secondary to capsule stretching.
- Management is by resection of symptomatic hemangiomas

*Hepatocellular Adenoma*

- Seen in women and strongly associated with oral contraceptive use
- Have pain and palpable abdominal mass
- Present with spontaneous rupture (mortality 9%)
- Hypervascular (angiography identifies blush)
- Biopsy to exclude malignancy
- Management with resection because of risk of rupture
- Avoid exogenous hormones and pregnancy

*Focal Nodular Hyperplasia*

- Women most common
- Symptoms similar to hepatic adenoma

- Rupture rare
- Management with resection

*Hemangioendothelioma*

- Benign liver tumor of children
- Malignant potential

## Malignant Hepatic Neoplasms

### *Hepatocellular Carcinoma*

- Most common primary malignant liver tumor

---

**FACT BOX 73**

The most common site of colorectal metastasis is the liver.

---

*Etiology*

- Chronic HBV
- Cirrhosis
- Hemochromatosis
- Schistosomiasis
- Aflatoxins

*Symptoms*

- Dull aching pain in RUQ
- Malaise
- Fever
- Jaundice

---

**FACT BOX 74**

Must have a bilirubin >3 before clinical jaundice is seen.

---

*Diagnosis*

- AFP is elevated in 70%–90% of cases.
- Ultrasound.
- CT.

*Treatment*

- Biopsy and exploration may be indicated to determine resectability.

## Hepatoblastoma

Most common primary malignant tumor of the liver in children.

*Symptoms*

- Abdominal distention
- Failure to thrive
- Hepatic failure

---

**FACT BOX 75**

Primary sclerosing cholangitis may be associated with inflammatory bowel disease (ulcerative colitis).

---

*Diagnosis*

- AFP
- CT scan

*Treatment*

- Surgical resection

## Angiosarcoma (Malignant Hemangioendothelioma)

Highly malignant tumor associated with past use of chemical agents including Thorotrast, vinyl chloride, and organochloride pesticides. Commonly spreads to spleen (80%). Surgical resection with <1 year survival.

## *Cholangiocarcinoma*

Arises from the bile duct epithelium. Etiologies include parasitic and primary sclerosing cholangitis. Treat with resection when feasible.

---

**FACT BOX 76**

Klatskin tumor is a tumor at the confluence of the hepatic ducts.

---

## Metastatic Neoplasms

### *Statistics*

- 0%–5% 5-year survival from colorectal metastasis without resection
- 30% 5-year survival for colorectal liver metastasis with resection

The liver is a common site of metastasis (second only to lymph nodes) for primary cancers secondary to hematogenous spread. More than 66% of colorectal cancers metastasize to the liver.

### *Labs*

- SGOT
- Alkaline phosphatase
- CEA

### *Radiology*

- Ultrasound is accurate screening scan.
- CT.

### *Treatment*

- Surgical resection is currently the only treatment modality that produced long-term survival advantage; ~20% are resectable at presentation.
- 30% 5-year survival.

- Cryosurgery.
- Radiofrequency ablation.
- Chemotherapy and radiation.
- Hepatic artery ligation (frequently is primary blood supply to tumors).

### Contraindications to Surgery

- Extrahepatic metastasis (other than solitary resectable lung mass).
- Portal nodal spread.
- Any number of metastases can be resected so long as adequate margins can be achieved while leaving sufficient residual tissue volume.
- Use of radiofrequency ablation (RFA) has provided a means of treating multiple masses, without extensive resections.

### Hepatic Resection

- Right hepatic lobectomy transects the liver through intralobular fissure.
- Left hepatic lobectomy same as above.
- Trisegmentectomy right lobe and median segment of left lobe.
- Left lateral segmentectomy removes segment to left of falciform ligament.
- Wedge resections.

Need to obtain 2-cm disease-free margins to minimize recurrence.

# 31

# Biliary

## Statistics

- 10% of population has gallstones.
- 15%–20% will develop symptoms.
- In 1% of biliary tract operations cancer is discovered.
- 8%–12% have CBD stones.
- <10% of asymptomatic gallstones will develop symptoms in 5 years.
- 10% can be visualized on AXR.

## Anatomy/Physiology

- Gallbladder holds 50 mL.
- *Hartmann's pouch*—infundibulum.
- *Triangle of Calot*—cystic duct, inferior border of liver, and common hepatic duct.
- Solubility of bile is based on concentrations of bile, cholesterol, and lecithin.

## Symptoms

- Right upper quadrant or epigastric pain
- Associated with meals and high-fat diets
- Nausea and vomiting
- Fever
- Jaundice

**Risk Factors**

- Female > male
- Age greater than 40
- Obesity
- Estrogen

*Biliary colic*—intermittent biliary pain that resolves after several hours to days. Caused by intermittent obstruction of the gallbladder by an impacted stone.

*Biliary dyskinesia*—poor motility and emptying of gallbladder. May be associated with acalculous cholecystitis. Ejection fraction <35%.

*Gallstone pancreatitis*—presence of gallstones and associated symptoms of pancreatitis including pain, enzyme elevations. Usually the result of obstruction of the pancreatic duct by a stone. Will need cholangiogram or ERCP to rule out CBD stones.

**Acute Cholecystitis**

*Etiology*

- Results from obstruction of the cystic duct
- Subsequent distention
- Lymphatic and venous congestion
- Inflammation

*Diagnosis*

- AXR—10% of stones can be seen
- Ultrasound—presence of gallstones, thickened gallbladder wall, dilated ducts
- Hepatobiliary iminodiacetic acid (HIDA) scan—failure of the gallbladder to fill with radioactive tag

*Treatment*

Cholecystectomy is indicated when the patient has had two or more episodes of biliary cholic or has developed acute cholecystitis.

- Resuscitation with IVF
- Antibiotics if acute cholecystitis (fever, N/V)

- NGT
- Laparoscopic cholecystectomy with conversion to open if needed (<5%)

## Gallstone Ileus

Small bowel obstruction secondary to impaction of a gallstone (>2.5 cm). Location is at the smallest diameter of the small bowel (ileocecal valve). Stone erodes through the GB wall and into the small bowel (duodenum most commonly).

- Usually occurs in elderly (>70).
- Diagnosis with AXR (40% have air in biliary tree), UGI.
- Treat with enterostomy and removal of the stone.

## Cholangitis

### *Etiology*

- Bacterial infection of the biliary tract.
- Most common cause is from obstruction.

### *Symptoms*

- Fever
- Right upper quadrant pain
- Jaundice

---

**FACT BOX 77**

Charcot's triad:
- Pain
- Fever
- Jaundice

---

## Reynold's Pentad

Cholangitis progresses to involve shock and mental status changes.
- Pain
- Fever

- Jaundice
- Mental status changes
- Shock

### Organisms

- *E. coli*
- *Klebsiella*
- *Enterococci*
- *B. fragilis*

### Diagnosis

- Elevated WBC, total bilirubin, and alk phos
- Ultrasound
- ERCP (endoscopic retrograde cholangiopancreatography)

### Management

Life threatening and requires immediate decompression of the biliary tree.

- ERCP—with stent placement
- PCTH (percutaneous transhepatic cholangiography)—externalized biliary drain placement

---

**FACT BOX 78**

Porcelain gallbladder from chronic cholecystitis is associated with cancer.
Courvoisier's gallbladder is a palpable nontender GB associated with pancreatic CA.

---

# 32

# Pancreas

**Anatomy**

- Duct of Wirsung is the main pancreatic duct.
- Duct of Santorini is accessory duct.

**Acute Pancreatitis**

Acute inflammation of the pancreas caused by autodigestion with
   pancreatic enzymes.
Most common cause is alcoholism and gallstones accounting for
   85% of cases.

*Symptoms*

- Epigastric pain
- Frequently radiating to back
- Nausea and vomiting
- Epigastric tenderness
- Decreased bowel sounds
- Fever
- Dehydration

*Differential Diagnosis*

- Gastritis or PUD
- Acute cholecystitis
- SBO

- Ruptured AAA
- Biliary colic
- Inferior MI

### Labs

- CBC, BMP
- LFT
- Amylase/lipase
- T&C
- ABG
- Ca

### Radiology

- Acute abdominal series (sentinel loop, colon cutoff, gallstones)
- Ultrasound
- CT for pseudocyst, phlegmon, abscess

### Treatment

- NPO
- NG
- IVF
- TPN
- $H_2$ blocker
- Demerol for pain control

#### Ranson Criteria

*3 at 48 hours indicates severe disease.*
   *At admission*
- >50 years old
- WBC >16K
- Glucose >200
- LDH >350
- SGOT >50

   *After 48 hours*
- BUN increase >5
- Hct fall >10%
- Serum Ca <8

- $pO_2$ <60
- Base deficit >4
- Fluid sequestration >6 L

| TABLE 32.1 Mortality by Ranson Criteria | |
|---|---|
| **Number of Criteria** | **% Mortality** |
| 0–2 | <5% |
| 3–4 | 20% |
| 5–6 | 40% |
| 7–8 | 99% |

## Chronic Pancreatitis

Chronic inflammation of the pancreas with destruction and fibrosis of pancreatic tissue. Most common etiology is EtOH.

### Symptoms

- Chronic waxing and waning abdominal pain with radiation to the back.

### Signs

- IDDM
- Steatorrhea
- Ascites
- Pleural effusion

### Differential Diagnosis

- Pancreatic cancer

### Labs

- Amylase, lipase

### Radiology

- CT
- KUB may identify calcifications in the pancreas.

## Treatment

- Analgesia
- Endocrine replacement
- Exocrine replacement (pancrelipase or pancreozymin)
- Bowel rest—TPN

## Surgical

*Puestow Operation*—Dilated chain of lakes duct treated by wide exposure of the duct and subsequent drainage by anastomosis of duct to defunctionalized loop of jejunum. Usually side to side.

*Distal Pancreatectomy*—Used for distal duct obstructive disease.

*Duval Operation*—Used for proximal duct obstructive disease. Resect the distal tail of pancreas and drain proximal pancreas retrograde into defunctionalized jejunal loop.

*Child Operation*—This is a 95% pancreatectomy.

*Splanchnicectomy*—Divides splanchnic nerves as palliation of severe refractory pain. It also eliminated visceral pain from other abdominal structures making diagnosis of disease difficult.

### Pancreatic Cancer

*Statistics*

- Fourth most common cause of cancer death in men in the United States
- 25,000 fatalities annually

---

**FACT BOX 79**

Most common site is head of pancreas.

---

## Symptoms

- Epigastric pain, weight loss, backache
- Pain radiating to back
- Painless jaundice
- Migratory thrombophlebitis

- *Courvoisier's Gallbladder* is the presence of a large nontender palpable gallbladder secondary to obstruction by the tumor.

The most common tumor location is the pancreatic head. Tumors produce weight loss and jaundice in 75% of patients. Tumors may be very large at time of presentation due to their retroperitoneal location

### Diagnosis

- Ultrasound
- ERCP
- CT
- CT-guided FNA
- Percutaneous transhepatic cholangiography. Useful to evaluate patients with possible obstructive jaundice.

### Treatment

Medical management is limited to chemotherapy, and surgery is indicated if the tumor is deemed resectable. Otherwise, chemotherapy and radiation are used primarily as palliative measures.

### Surgery

The tumor is determined to be resectable if there are no metastases, does not involve the porta hepatis, and has not spread to the liver.

*Pancreatoduodenectomy (Whipple Procedure)*

- Cholecystectomy
- Truncal vagotomy
- Antrectomy
- Pancreatoduodenectomy
- Choledochojejunostomy
- Pancreatojejunostomy
- Gastrojejunostomy

*Total Pancreatectomy.* May offer advantage by removing multicentric tumors that occur in up to 40% of patients.

*Palliative Surgery Includes:*

- Relief of biliary tract obstruction
- Gastric outlet obstruction (gastrojejunostomy, choledochoje-junostomy)
- Stents for obstructive jaundice

Chemotherapy has a 20%–25% response rate.

### *Prognosis*

- <1% 5-year survival (most within the first year).
- <6 month for unresectable tumors.
- 10% with resectable tumors and subsequent surgery survive 5 years.
- <10% of pancreatic adenocarcinomas are resectable at time of diagnosis.

# 33

# Hernias

**Anatomy**

- Internal inguinal ring formed by transversalis fascia.
- External inguinal ring formed by external oblique aponeurosis.
- Anterior wall formed by external oblique aponeurosis.
- Inferior wall formed by inguinal ligament.
- Roof is formed by internal oblique and transversus abdominis muscles forming the conjoint tendon.
- Posterior wall is formed by transversalis fascia and aponeurosis.
- Structures in the spermatic cord—testicular and cremasteric arteries, ilioinguinal and genital branch of genitofemoral nerves, sympathetics, pampiniform plexus, vas deferens, process vaginalis.

*Etiology*

Inguinal hernias most commonly are indirect and are the result of a patent process vaginalis and increases in intra-abdominal pressure. Always look for the following in a patient with a hernia of any type:
- COPD
- BPH or prostate cancer
- Constipation
- Intra-abdominal neoplastic disease

---

FACT BOX **80**

Hesselbach's triangle:
- Inferior epigastric vv.
- Inguinal ligament
- Lateral border of rectus abdominis

---

## Types

- Reducible—hernia returns to its normal space.
- Incarcerated—hernia trapped and does not return to normal space.
- Strangulated—hernia is incarcerated with compromised blood supply.

## Treatment

*Surgical Repair*

*High ligation of hernia sack*—pediatric inguinal hernia almost always indirect and 75% on right.

*Bassini* involves transversalis fascia, conjoint tendon sutured to the inguinal ligament.

*McVay's (Cooper's ligament repair)* transversalis fascia to Cooper's ligament.

*Shouldice* repair like Bassini except transversalis fascia is divided longitudinally and imbricated upon itself in two layers.

---

FACT BOX **81**

Most common . . .
Inguinal hernia is indirect.
Inguinal hernia in male or female is indirect.

---

## Hernia Quick Draw

*Indirect Hernia*—lateral to inferior epigastric vessels
*Direct Hernia*—medial to inferior epigastric vessels
*Richter's Hernia*—incarcerated or strangulated hernia involving only one side of the bowel wall (knuckle of bowel)

189

*Littrés Hernia*—involves a Meckel's diverticulum
*Spigelian Hernia*—through the linea semilunaris
*Pantaloon Hernia*—passes both medially and laterally to epigastric vessels

# 34

# Thyroid

**Thyroid Carcinoma**

*Statistics*

- 70% papillary.
- 20% of cold nodules are malignant.
- 5% of FNA for false negatives.
- 10% of palpable solitary nodules are malignant, 20% if cold.

*Anatomy: Arterial Supply*

- Superior thyroid artery
- Inferior thyroid artery
- Thyroid IMA artery

*Nerves*

*Recurrent Laryngeal* (motor to true vocal cords)

- Damage results in hoarseness (unilateral damage), vocal cord paralysis, and airway obstruction (bilateral).

*Superior Laryngeal* (motor to cricothyroid and sensory to supraglotic pharynx)

- Damage results in weak voice (bad for opera singers).

## History

- Very young or very old
- Previous neck irradiation
- Hypofunctioning or nonfunctioning nodule
- Family history of thyroid cancer
- Familial adenomatous polyposis (FAP)
- MEN syndromes (IIa and IIb)

## Pathology

### Papillary

- 60%–70%
- Young women
- Psammoma bodies

### Follicular

- 15%–20%
- Hematogenous spread (lung and bone)

### Medullary

- Produces calcitonin
- Associated with MEN II

### Anaplastic

- 10%–15%
- Worst prognosis

Benign tumors include:
- Follicular adenoma
- Adenomatous goiter
- Thyroiditis

---

**FACT BOX 82**

A history of neck irradiation increases the chances of either papillary or follicular thyroid cancer.

---

### Diagnosis

- Thyroid function tests frequently not helpful
- Ultrasound to identify if cystic/solid, multiple/solitary
- FNA
- Radionuclide scan usually not needed

### Surgical Indications

- Cancer
- Questionable lesion
- Local symptoms—dysphagia, airway impingement

### Surgery

*Lobectomy*

- Papillary carcinomas
- Leaves thyroid tissue
- Risk of recurrence—20%–60% are multicentric carcinomas

*Total Thyroidectomy*

- Removes all gross thyroid tissue.
- Residual can be ablated with $^{131}$iodine.
- Medullary carcinoma requires a total thyroidectomy and central neck dissection.

### Postoperative Treatment

- Give exogenous thyroid hormone to suppress TSH (accelerated CA growth).
- Whole body radioiodine scan to identify mets.
- Doxorubicin for tumors without iodine uptake.

## Thyrotoxicosis

### Graves' Disease

- Exophthalmos
- Diffuse goiter
- Pretibial myxedema

## Thyroiditis

- Subacute (DeQuervain)—usually viral cause
- Acute—inflammation of gland following recent bacterial infection
- Chronic (Hashimoto)—autoimmune

## Multinodular Goiter

> **FACT BOX 83**
>
> Iodine is used preoperatively to block thyroid output and decrease vascularity (Wolf-Chaikoff effect).

## Treatment

- Antithyroid medication (propylthiouracil, beta blockers)
- Radioactive iodine to ablate hyperfunctioning tissue

## Surgery

- *Subtotal thyroidectomy* leaving posterior thyroid intact to preserve parathyroids and minimize injury to recurrent laryngeal nerve

> **FACT BOX 84**
>
> *Struma ovari* is thyroid tissue in ovarian teratoma.

## Medical Management

- Propranolol blocks peripheral hypermetabolic manifestations.
- Propylthiouracil (PTU) or methimazole $\times$ 8–10 days with iodine preoperatively.

## Thyroid Storm

Thyroid storm is the hypersecretion in hyperthyroid patients secondary to stressors such as surgery. Can lead to high-output cardiac failure, hypertension, hypermetabolic state and death. Presents with hyperpyrexia, tachycardia, irritability, nausea, vomiting.

### Treatment

- Cooling
- Volume resuscitation
- Steroids (hydrocortisone 100 mg)
- Beta blockade (propranolol 1–2 mg, 50–100 mcg/min IV drip)
- Sodium iodide
- Glucose monitoring

## Hyperparathyroid

### Statistics

- 85% are single adenoma.
- 85% of adenomas are found in normal locations.
- 40% are located in thymic tongue.

### Anatomy

- Upper pair from fourth brachial arch and lower pair from third.
- Superior thyroid artery supplies all four glands.

Primary hyperparathyroidism presents with one of three histologic subtypes.
- Adenoma
- Hyperplasia
- Carcinoma

### Symptoms

The majority (70%) of patients are asymptomatic at presentation and are discovered secondary to routine labs for other medical problems. The classic presentation of hypercalcemic state otherwise prevails in 20% of patients.
- Stones—nephrolithiasis
- Bones—bone pain, muscle ache, arthralgias
- Groans—secondary PUD (increased gastrin), pancreatitis
- Psychiatric overtones—fatigue, depression, irritability in 40% of patients

## *Diagnosis*

- Serum PTH
- Ca

---

**FACT BOX 85**

Hyperparathyroid triad:
- Hypercalcemia
- Hypophosphatemia
- Increased urinary $Ca^{2+}$ and $PO_4$

---

**FACT BOX 86**

Iatrogenic causes of hypercalcemia:
    Thiazide diuretics
    TUMS or other antacids with $Ca^{2+}$

---

## *Treatment*

- Resuscitation with NS
- Forced diuresis with furosemide
- Etidronate 7.5 mg/kg qd $\times$ 3 days, then 5–20 mg/kg po qd
- Mithramycin 25 mcg/kg over 4 hours

## *Surgery*

*Parathyroidectomy*

- Resection of the adenoma with preservation of remaining glands
- Resection of all four glands in hyperplasia with autotransplantation to forearm muscle

FACT BOX **87**

Hyperparathyroid:
- Most common cause is adenoma.
- Most common cause of secondary hyper-parathyroidism is dialysis for CRF.
- Most common cause of hypercalcemia in hospital patients is bone metastasis.

# 35

# Adrenal

**Anatomy**

Three functional layers:
- Glomerulosa—aldosterone
- Fasciculata—cortisol
- Reticularis—testosterone, androgens
  (GFR–ACT)

**Hyperaldosteronism (Conn Syndrome)**

*Etiology*

- Adenoma
- Hyperplasia
- Carcinoma
- Renovascular disease

*Symptoms*

- Hypertension
- Cramps
- Polydipsia, polyuria

*Diagnosis*

- Hypernatremia, hypokalemia, decreased renin

- Na loading with 24-hour urinary aldosterone determination
- CT/MRI localization

### Treatment

- Spironolactone 25–50 mg PO qd/bid
- Correct hypokalemia

### Surgery

- Unilateral adrenalectomy

## Cushing Syndrome

Results from excessive cortisol production. ACTH stimulus from pituitary adenoma or ectopic source.

### Signs and Symptoms

- HTN
- Hyperglycemia
- Fatigue
- Easy bruising
- Truncal obesity
- Buffalo hump
- Purple striae

---

**FACT BOX 88**

*Nelson's syndrome*—secondary to bilateral adrenalectomy leading to hypersecretion of ACTH and subsequent hyperpigmentation and pituitary enlargement

---

### Diagnosis

Dexamethasone suppression test

ACTH = no change

- *Cushing syndrome*—hyperfunctioning adenoma/hyperplasia

ACTH = normal to elevated
- *Cushing's disease*—excessive production of ACTH by pituitary

ACTH = elevated
- Ectopic ACTH–secreting tumor

### Treatment

*Cushing's Disease* (pituitary adenoma)—excision of adenoma

*Cushing's Syndrome*

*Medical*
- Mitotane—selectively atrophies and necroses the zona fasciculata

*Surgical*
- Adrenalectomy—unilateral for adenoma/cancer or bilateral for hyperplasia
- Treat underlying source of exogenous ACTH (bronchial carcinoid, small cell carcinoma)

### Postoperative

Need to give supplemental steroids.
- Hydrocortisone 100 mg IV preop and in recovery, then q6h and taper
- Maintenance with prednisone 5 mg PO in the morning and 2.5 PO in the evening

# 36

# Pheochromocytoma

Pheochromocytoma is an adrenal medulla tumor with hyper-secretion of catecholamines. It is located along the sympathetic ganglia, adrenal gland, or bladder.

## *Statistics*

Rule of 10
- 10% bilateral
- 10% malignant
- 10% extra-adrenal
- 10% in children
- 80% bilateral in MEN II

---

**FACT BOX 89**

Pheochromocytoma triad:
- Hypertension
- Palpitations
- Diaphoresis

---

## *Symptoms*

- Hypertension
- Headache
- Diaphoresis
- Palpitations

### *Diagnosis*

- Urinary catecholamines—vanillylmandelic acid (VMA), meta-nephrine, and normetanephrine
- CT/US/MRI to localize tumor
- $^{131}I$ MIBG (iodine-131 metaiodobenzylguanidine)

### *Preoperative Management*

- Phenoxybenzamine 10 mg PO bid 10–14 days preop
- Propranolol 40 mg PO bid to control peripheral effects (always give alpha before beta)

---

**FACT BOX 90**

Always give alpha blockade before beta blockade; otherwise unopposed alpha constriction with loss of beta$_2$ vasodilatation would result.

---

**FACT BOX 91**

Pheochromocytoma:
- Most common ectopic location at organ of Zuckerkandl near aortic arch.
- Elevated norepinephrine indicates extra-adrenal location as these sites lack enzyme to methylate norepi to epi.
- Hypertensive crisis with urination suggests a bladder pheochromocytoma.

# 37

# Melanoma

## Statistics

- 1% of all cancer deaths
- Eighth most common cancer in the United States
- 1.3% lifetime risk of developing melanoma

## Risks

- Sun exposure
- Caucasian
- Fair skin
- History of sunburn as child

## Physical Characteristics

- Change in size
- Color
- Shape
- Consistency
- Pain
- Adenopathy

```
┌─────────────────────────────────────────────────────────┐
│ ┌──────────────────┐                                      │
│ │ FACT BOX 92      │                                      │
│ └──────────────────┘                                      │
│   ABCD:                                                    │
│   Asymmetry                    Color variation             │
│   Border irregularity          Diameter >6 mm              │
│                                                            │
└─────────────────────────────────────────────────────────┘
```

**Diagnosis**

- Excisional biopsy
- Incisional biopsy with frozen sections if large lesion

**Pathology**

- Superficial spreading
- Nodular
- Lentigo maligna
- Acral lentiginous

**Staging**

- LFT
- Alkaline phosphatase
- CXR
- Physical exam (attention to nodal basins, mental status, bone pain)

**Treatment**

*Wide local excision with margins*
- In general for each 1-mm depth of invasion give 1-cm margin with excision (2 cm max).
- In situ 0.5-mm margins.

*Sentinel node biopsy*—false negative rates <2%, successfully identifies micrometastasis to nodal basins. If sentinel node is positive completion node dissection can be done.
*Elective lymph node dissection (ELND)*—for lesions between 0.76 mm and 4 mm thick.

*Adjuvant therapy* includes regional hyperthermic perfusion (high-dose chemotherapy at high temperatures).
*Immunotherapy* (IFN gamma) for cutaneous metastasis.

**Staging**

The most accepted staging system resides in the Breslow. This is a measure of the depth of invasion.

**TABLE 37.1**
**Breslow Staging**

| Stage | Breslow Depth | Mortality at 5 Years |
| --- | --- | --- |
| T1 | <0.76 mm | 10% |
| T2 | 0.76–1.5 mm | 15% |
| T3 | 1.51–4.0 mm | 50% |
| T4 | >4 mm | 75% |

The Clark level is based on the level of invasion:
- I  confined to epidermis
- II  invades papillary dermis
- III  fills papillary dermis
- IV  invades reticular dermis
- V  invades subcutaneous fat

# 38

# Trauma

## Statistics

- 150,000 annual deaths in United States.
- 33% of all hospital admissions are trauma related.
- 50% of deaths occur at scene.

In general, the evaluation of a trauma patient differs from that of a normal surgical patient in that it requires an urgent, orderly approach. The trauma room can be a very confusing place, and it is up to the team leader (trauma surgeon) to maintain order. The primary survey identifies life-threatening injuries and should take only 30 to 60 seconds.

## Primary Survey Targets

- Airway—Establish a patent airway.
- Breathing—Ensure that both lungs are being ventilated.
- Circulation—Check for peripheral pulses, and apply direct pressure to bleeds.
- Disability—Assess the neurological status of the patient briefly.
- Exposure—Fully expose the patient and examine all areas for injury.

Do not move to the next step until urgent problems are solved (i.e., airway, breathing, circulation).

## Primary Survey

*Airway and c-spine*—Chin lift and jaw thrust without hyperextension or flexion. Assume c-spine trauma with injuries above the clavicle.

*Breathing*—Observe chest movement, auscultate, bag mask, intubate as needed. Search for tension pneumothorax, open/flail chest.

*Circulation*—Cardiac output evaluation of pulse, skin color, capillary refill.

- Radial = systolic >80
- Femoral = systolic >70
- Carotid = systolic >60

Identify and control exsanguinating hemorrhage in the primary survey. Direct pressure, pneumatic splints. Look for occult bleeds into abdomen, chest, pelvis.

*Disability*—Brief neuro exam to evaluate the level of consciousness (alert, vocal stimulus, painful stimulus, unresponsive). Ask patient's name; ask him or her to squeeze hands and wiggle toes.

*Expose*—Completely undress the patient and roll patient to look for injuries to back.

## Resuscitation

- Oxygen
- IV (2 large bore and start 2 L LR)
- Type and cross
- CBC, Chem 18, amylase, PT/PTT, HCG
- UA
- Vitals
- Foley placement (must rule out urethral transection blood at meatus, high-riding prostate)
- NG tube if no cribriform plate fracture (blunt head trauma, nonclotting blood from nose, ears)

---

**FACT BOX 93**

Most important lab in trauma is the T&C.

---

**FACT BOX 94**

The 6 tubes of Wrightson:
Make sure there is a tube in every orifice if
required.
- Endotracheal tube
- Large-bore IV (2)
- NG tube
- Foley catheter
- Chest tube

---

## Ultrasound (FAST Scan)

Assess four windows for free fluid.
- Subxyphoid
- Splenorenal recess
- Hepatorenal recess
- Suprapubic

## Trauma Films

- *C-spine film*—obtain cross-table lateral or swimmer's view of c-spine with all 7 cervical vertebrae visible. Must see through to T1 for adequate films.
- *Chest*—look for evidence of pneumothorax (remember PNX is a clinical diagnosis), hemothorax, fractures.
- *Pelvic x-rays*—fractures.

## Secondary Survey

*Head*

- Pupil size/equal, fundal hemorrhages, lens dislocation, conjunctival hemorrhages, penetrating injuries
- Ecchymosis around ears (Battle's sign) and periorbital ecchymosis (raccoon eyes) suggest basilar skull fracture

*Maxillofacial*

- Not necessary to treat emergently. Priority is protection of the airway and to document any midfacial fractures or instability.

*C-spine and Neck*

- Palpate for deformities and/or crepitus. Assume patients with face trauma have c-spine injury. Penetrating trauma through the platysma should not be probed in the ER but evaluated with arteriography, bronchoscopy, esophagoscopy.

*Chest*

- Sucking chest wound, flail chest.
- Palpate ribs and clavicles.
- Listen for breath sounds bilaterally and heart sounds.

*Abdomen*

- Examine for signs of trauma, ecchymosis, seatbelt sign.
- Penetrating injuries.
- Paradoxical retractions.
- Close observation but if patient is not alert or has equivocal findings obtain a CT with oral/IV contrast.

*Rectum*

- Blood in the lumen
- High-riding prostate
- Pelvic fracture
- Integrity of rectal wall
- Sphincter tone

*Fractures*

- Examine extremities for contusions or deformities.
- Palpate bones for crepitation or tenderness.
- Inward compression of anterior superior iliac spines and anterior to posterior compression of symphysis pubis can identify pelvic fractures.
- Check all peripheral pulses.

*Neurological*

- Motor and sensory information, pupils, Glasgow Coma Scale Score

| TABLE 38.1 Glasgow Coma Scale | | |
|---|---|---|
| **Eye Opening** | **Motor Response** | **Vocal Response** |
| 4 Spontaneous | 6 Obeys commands | 5 Oriented ×3 |
| 3 Opens to command | 5 Localizes pain | 4 Confused |
| 2 Opens to pain | 4 Withdraws from pain | 3 Inappropriate |
| 1 None | 3 Flexion with pain | 2 Incomprehensible |
| | 2 Extension with pain | 1 None |
| | 1 None | |

## History

*AMPLE*—Allergies, medications, past medical history, last meal, events related to injury.

*Re-evaluate* the patient for new signs and symptoms, vitals, and urine output.

---

FACT BOX **95**

This book has a Glasgow Coma Score of 3.

---

## Thoracic Trauma

### Primary Survey

ABCs

Life-threatening injuries in primary survey
- Airway obstruction
- Tension pneumothorax
- Complete collapse of the affected lung, mediastinal shift to opposite side, hypotension

**Tension Pneumothorax**

Causes include blunt/penetrating trauma, excessive PEEP (>20), spontaneous.

*Physical Exam*—Tracheal deviation, respiratory distress, unilateral absence of the breath sounds, distended neck veins, tympanic to percussion over the affected side.

*Treatment*—Large-bore angiocath in second intercostal space mid-clavicular line. Chest tube into fourth intercostal space anterior to midaxillary line.

---

FACT BOX **96**

Tension pneumothorax is a clinical diagnosis. It is not diagnosed by CXR.

---

## *Open Pneumothorax*

Results from penetrating injuries with air escaping into the wound with each respiratory effort.

Treatment with occlusive dressing taped on three sides. If possible chest tube placed away from the wound and surgical repair.

## *Massive Hemothorax*

Loss of 1500 cc or more of blood into the chest. Cause is penetrating trauma to systemic or pulmonary vessels or blunt trauma.

*Physical Exam*—Shock with absence of breath sounds and dullness to percussion on one side.

*Treatment*—IVF, blood, chest tube at nipple level anterior to midaxillary line. Patients will require a thoracotomy. Indications for thoracotomy:
- >1000 mL blood out chest tube initially
- >200 mL/h for 4 hours

## *Flail Chest*

Trauma with multiple rib fractures and underlying lung contusion.

*Physical Exam*—Multiple rib fractures and paradoxical respirations

*Treatment*—With mechanical ventilation, pain relief (epidural if T&L spines clear)

Lung contusion will worsen over 12–36 hours and slowly resolve. Careful with IVF as the pulmonary contusion flowers.

### Cardiac Tamponade

Effusion (blood) in pericardial sac causing impaired cardiac output. Penetrating injuries, blunt injuries.

*Physical Exam*

- Hypotension
- Distant heart sounds
- JVD

---

**FACT BOX 97**

*Beck's triad—Tamponade:*
- Distended neck veins
- Distant heart sounds
- Hypotension

---

*Treatment*—Pericardiocentesis by subxyphoid approach with 16-gauge needle angiocath. Definitive treatment is pericardiotomy with pericardial window.

### Secondary Survey

Potential lethal injuries in secondary survey.

*Pulmonary contusion*—Respiratory insufficiency develops over a period of time (12–36 hours).
Treatment with mechanical ventilation.

*Traumatic Aortic Rupture*—MVA, fall from height.

*Radiology*—Widened mediastinum, obliteration of aortic knob, deviation of trachea to right, pleural cap, elevation of right mainstem bronchus, depression of left mainstem bronchus.

- *Widened mediastinum*—ominous finding on plain CXR. Suggests great vessel injury (aortic transection most commonly). If not certain, a 72-inch CRX or CT of mediastinum can help in diagnosis. If in doubt, arch aortogram.

*Tracheal Injuries*—Penetrating or blunt injuries. Fracture of larynx, hoarseness, subcutaneous emphysema, crepitus, noisy breathing, complete airway obstruction.
*Diagnosis*—Laryngoscopy, bronchoscopy
*Treatment*—Surgery as definitive treatment

*Bronchial Injuries*—Signs are hemoptysis, sub-q emphysema, mediastinal shift, persistent pneumothorax or air leak after chest tube or thoracotomy.

*Esophageal Trauma*—Signs are left pneumothorax or hemothorax without rib fracture. Mediastinal air, particulate matter in chest tube.
*Diagnosis*—Gastrografin swallow or esophagoscopy
*Treatment*—NPO, surgical repair, drainage

*Traumatic Diaphragmatic Hernia*—Blunt trauma.
*Diagnosis*—CXR shows NG tube in chest, elevated left hemidiaphragm
*Treatment*—Repair of diaphragmatic rent

*Myocardial Contusion*—Results from blunt trauma.
*Diagnosis*—Elevated CPK, ECG abnormalities
*Treatment*—Admit to unit with continuous monitoring

### Indications for Chest Tube

- Pneumothorax
- Hemothorax
- Suspected severe lung injury

### Abdominal Trauma

The most important point to remember is to identify an intra-abdominal injury and get the unstable patient to the OR.

### Primary Survey

- Look at the anterior and posterior walls of the abdomen, flanks, lower chest, buttocks, and perineum. Contusions, abrasions, lacerations, and penetrating wounds should be identified.
- Listen for the presence or absence of bowel sounds. Feel for guarding and tenderness.

#### Areas to Evaluate

*Intrathoracic abdomen*—Spleen, stomach, liver, diaphragm all may be involved in rib fractures, sternal injury, seatbelt injury. Adjunctive studies include x-ray, Gastrografin swallow, CT.

---

**FACT BOX 98**

Most common blunt intra-abdominal injury is spleen laceration.

---

*True Abdomen*—Small and large bowel with signs of increasing abdominal pain, decreasing bowel sounds, positive FAST scan, free air. Gross blood on rectal exam.

*Retroperitoneal Abdomen*—Difficult to assess. Retroperitoneal hematomas diagnosed best with CT. Kidney and ureters examined via IVP and may show hemorrhage or extravasation of urine. Duodenal injury is suspected by unusual air patterns in the RUQ or extravasation of Gastrografin. Pancreatic, duodenal, and small bowel injuries may be identified with elevated amylase. Vascular injuries identified by hemorrhage, loss of pulses, hypotension, ischemia, bruit.

*Rectal Exam*—Look at the perineum; feel for sphincter tone, integrity of rectal wall, position of prostate, mobility of prostate; look at exam finger for blood.

*Vaginal*—Injuries from penetrating or blunt trauma. Open pelvic fractures may be identified by tears or lacerations of vaginal wall. A careful pelvic exam may identify these injuries.

214

## Types of Injuries

*Penetrating*—Wounds on abdomen, lower chest, flanks and buttocks. Result in hemorrhage from major vessel or solid organ or perforation of bowel. Do not remove the object. Bleeding is evident and manifested by increasing distention, rigidity, quiet abdomen, shock, abdominal pain.

*Blunt Injuries*—Require a high index of suspicion. Look, listen, and feel. Ultrasound is a useful screening device for free fluid.

## Treatment

*Labs*

- CBC, type and cross, PT/PTT, amylase, hCG, 2 large-bore IVs.

*Tubes*

- NG—therapeutic as it relieves and prevents gastric distention, removes gastric contents, and helps to prevent possible aspiration. Diagnostic of bleeds. Contraindicated in cribriform plate fracture.
- Foley—Therapeutic in monitoring urine output, urine specimen. Diagnostic for gross hematuria, IVP, and cystourethrogram as indicated. Precautions as rectal exam must be performed first to rule out fractured pelvis and urethral injuries. Contraindicated if meatal blood, scrotal or perianal hematoma, or high-riding prostate. Suprapubic catheter is alternate means of bladder drainage.

*Radiology*

- Upright chest or left lateral decubitus film to detect free air, fractures, loss of psoas shadow or foreign bodies.
- Supine film of abdomen for retroperitoneal air, gross organ injury, foreign body.
- CT is the best diagnostic test for blunt abdominal injury to identify liver, spleen, renal injury as well as free fluid in the abdomen.

## Diagnostic Peritoneal Lavage (DPL)

CT and US have replaced DPL in recent years. It is still performed in many situations when CT/US are not readily available, or hemodynamic instability with a positive physical exam in light of a negative CT. Small incidence of complications, beneficial for occult injury in blunt trauma, not reliable for retroperitoneal bleeds.

### Indications

Patients with history of blunt abdominal trauma who have altered level of consciousness, intoxication, or spinal trauma. Patients who have unexplained hypovolemia following multiple trauma, equivocal exam, lower rib fracture, lumbar spine fracture (a supraumbilical approach may be employed with pelvic fracture to avoid false positives). Patients who have suspected abdominal injuries after sustaining trauma to the lower chest, flank, or buttocks. Patients who have sustained severe trauma but have negative exam and will be unavailable for continued monitoring (i.e., in OR to repair fractures, etc.).

### Contraindications

*Absolute.* History of multiple abdominal operations, obvious indications for exploratory laparotomy.

*Relative.* Pregnancy, open technique above the uterus may be used.

### Complications

- Abdominal wall bleeding giving a false positive
- Abdominal bleeding requiring operative repair
- Perforation of intra-abdominal or retroperitoneal organs
- Peritonitis resulting in subsequent alterations of the physical exam

### Interpretation

- 10 cc of grossly bloody aspirate
- >100 K RBC

- \>500 WBC
- Spun Hct >2
- Presence of bile, bacteria, fecal, or vegetable matter.

Negative DPL does not rule out retroperitoneal injuries to the pancreas, duodenum, GU, aorta, vena cava, or diaphragm.

## GU Injuries

### History

Blunt trauma to the abdomen, lower chest, flank, genitalia, perineum, associated with hematuria, decreased urine output, abdominal or flank mass, swelling of the genitalia. These individuals are prone to arterial intimal tears and thrombosis and, in children, avulsion of the ureter at the ureteropelvic junction. Penetrating wounds of the abdomen, flank, genitalia, or pelvis.

*Physical Exam*—Hematoma or fractured ribs 10–12, discoloration, penetrating wound or mass in the flank, lower abdominal mass or tenderness, genital swelling or discoloration, inability to void, blood at the urethral meatus.

*Radiology*—IVP and cystourethrogram to evaluate the upper and lower tracts.

### Pelvic Fractures

Should alert you to other serious injuries in the chest, spine, and abdomen. It should be suspected in patient with unexplained shock following blunt trauma and can lead to exsanguinating hemorrhage. Signs of pain, crepitation, abnormal motion. Pelvic fractures can result in significant blood loss.

*Radiology*—Plain pelvic films or CT.

*Treatment*—External or open fixation. If continued bleeding arteriography with embolization of active bleeding vessels may be necessary.

# 39

# Burns

## Assessment

- ABCs.
- Vitals.
- Extent of burn (body surface area and depth).
- Stop the burning process.
- Remove all clothing.

### *Primary Survey*

*Airway and Breathing*

Signs of inhalational injury should be sought as they may lead to airway obstruction in 24–48 hours. These signs are
- Facial burns
- Singeing of the eyebrows and nasal hair
- Carbon deposits and acute inflammatory changes in the oropharynx
- Carbonaceous sputum
- History of impaired mentation
- Confinement in a burning environment

Endotracheal intubation and mechanical ventilation should be initiated if signs of airway burn present. All patients should initially receive supplemental oxygen.

*Circulation*

- If the patient has burns >20 BSA, he or she will need fluid resuscitation.
- Two large-bore catheters should be placed in a peripheral vein.
- Upper extremities are preferred. It is OK to place an IV into a burned area.
- Ringer's lactate should be infused according to urine output.
  - Initial resuscitation by the *Parkland formula*:
    - Amount of LR required = 2–4 mL × BSA × kg (given in the first 24 hours with 1/2 given in the first 8 hours and the remaining half given over 16 hours. For children, use this formula plus maintenance).

As always urine output should be:
- 1 cc/kg/h in children
- 30–50 cc/h in adults

*History*

AMPLET
- Allergies
- Medications
- Past medical history
- Last meal
- Events related to incident
- Tetanus status

*Physical Exam*

Assess the depth and extent of the burn:
- 1st degree is red and painful like that of a sunburn. Involves epidermis only.
- 2nd degree is red, with swelling, pain, blistering. Epidermis with varying degrees of dermis.
- 3rd degree is dark and leathery or white, surface is usually dry and painless. All layers of skin.

| TABLE 39.1 BSA Rule of 9s | |
| --- | --- |
| Burn Area | % Total Body Surface Area |
| Head and neck | 9 |
| Arm | 9 |
| Whole leg | 18 |
| Anterior chest abdomen | 18 |
| Back and buttocks | 18 |
| Perineum | 1 |

Patient's hand is ~1% BSA.

*Extremities*—Assess the pulses, cyanosis, paresthesias. In the case of insufficient flow from a circumferential burn, escharotomy should be performed.

*Chest*—A circumferential burn of the chest can impair respiratory excursion and bilateral midaxillary escharotomy incisions should be considered to improve respiratory function.

*Treatment*

- Place an NG tube for any patient with N/V or BSA >25%, also place Foley catheter.
- Pain management as needed.
- *Wound Care*—Apply fresh laundered linens to deflect air currents, break blisters, debride loose devitalized tissue. Topical antibiotics are applied (Bacitracin, Silvadene, sulfamylon, silver nitrate).

*Labs*

- CBC
- ABG
- BMP
- Carboxyhemoglobin

*Special Burns*

*Chemical Burns*—Alkali is more serious that acid. Irrigate with water immediately for 20–30 minutes. Burns of the eye require continuous flushing for 8 hours.

*Electrical Burns*—ECG to evaluate cardiac function. Initiate IV fluids to maintain urine output of 100 cc/h because of myoglobinuria. Check urine myoglobin q8h or until three negative results. Mannitol (25 g, then 12.5 g/L of fluid) and bicarbonate to produce brisk diureses and alkalize urine.

FACT BOX 99

Hyponatremia is associated with silver nitrate administration.
Neutropenia is associated with silvadene administration.

# 40

# Vascular Surgery

**Peripheral Vascular Disease**

*Statistics*

- 50% of patients with claudication have occlusion at Hunter's canal.
- >30% have severe coexisting CAD.

*Risk Factors*

- Smoking
- Diabetes
- Hypertension
- Hyperlipidemia
- Arteriosclerosis

Patients with peripheral vascular disease likely have coronary artery disease.

---

**FACT BOX 100**

The most common cause of death for a patient with PVD is MI.

---

### Site of Stenosis

- Bifurcations.
- Adductor canal (Hunter's canal) is most common site for PVD.

### Symptoms

*Claudication*—Leg or calf pain with exertion. Claudication is reproducible at constant distance and is relieved with rest

*Rest Pain*—Pain that is not relieved with rest. Patients will commonly say it wakes them at night and they sleep with their leg off the side of the bed for better comfort.

*LeRiche Syndrome*—Iliac vessel disease resulting in butt and thigh claudication and impotence.

### Workup

- Ankle-brachial index (ABI)
- Arteriography
- Digital subtraction angiography

**TABLE 40.1**
**Ankle-Brachial Index**

| Symptoms | ABI |
| --- | --- |
| Normal | 1.0 |
| Claudication | 0.6–0.8 |
| Rest pain | 0.3–0.5 |

Calcified arteries increase the ABI, seen commonly with DM.

### Chronic Peripheral Vascular Disease

Peripheral vascular disease (PVD) with chronic progression. Occlusive atherosclerotic lesions mainly in the lower extremities. The presentation is also progressive:

- Intermittent claudication
- Rest pain
- Sensory motor loss
- Tissue ischemia and necrosis

223

*Intermittent claudication* presents as crampy pain in the lower extremities that
- Occurs at specific distance
- Is relieved by rest
- Is reproducible

The symptoms are present distal to the site of obstruction or arterial narrowing.

### Management

Control of intermittent claudication is best achieved by lifestyle modifications. This includes:
- Exercise program
- Cessation of smoking
- Pentoxifylline is used with variable success. It reduces blood viscosity by decreasing plasma fibrinogen and platelet aggregation.

### Prognosis

*Claudication* is a strong indicator of atherosclerotic disease with the most common cause of death being heart disease. Patients with claudication can be divided into three groups based on the natural history of the disease.
- 1/3 continue with same symptoms.
- 1/3 progress to rest pain.
- 1/3 lose the limb.

*Rest pain* is the result of severely compromised arterial flow to the extremity. It presents as an intense pain with exacerbation when the leg is elevated and relief with the limb in a dependent position such as hanging off the side of a bed.

### Indications for Surgery

- Severe claudication affecting normal activities
- Ischemia
- Peripheral artery emboli
- Impotence

---

FACT BOX **101**

In general, all PVD is treated in one of four ways:
- Observation, lifestyle modification
- Bypass
- Endarterectomy
- Angioplasty

---

## Surgery

The procedures below make use of an autologous saphenous vein graft or synthetic (Dacron, Goretex) graft. Vein grafts tend to have better patency rates as compared to synthetic materials.

*Femoropopliteal Bypass*
- 80% 5-year patency with 90% limb salvage

*Femorotibial Bypass*
- 70% 5-year patency with 80% limb salvage
- 20% 1-year patency with Dacron or PTFE grafts (avoid synthetic grafts below the knee)

*Profundoplasty* is the repair of the origin of the profunda femoris artery.

*Amputation* is indicated for patients when reconstructive surgery is not feasible.
- Rehabilitation rate is ~70% for below the knee amputations (BKA) and as low as 10% for above the knee amputations.

## Acute Arterial Insufficiency

Acute occlusion of a vessel may occur because of a thrombus or embolus. The most common site affected by embolism is at the bifurcation. In the lower extremity the most common site is the bifurcation of the common femoral into the superficial and deep femoral arteries.

### Etiology—Source of Emboli
- Heart (60%) secondary to atrial fibrillation, mural thrombi

- Aortic or proximal vessel
- Rarely patent foramen ovale
- Rheumatic valve diagnosis

---

**FACT BOX 102**

Irreversible tissue damage occurs after 6 hours of occlusion.

---

### Signs of Acute Arterial Occlusion (6 Ps)

- Pain
- Paralysis
- Paresthesia
- Pallor
- Pulseless
- Polar

---

**FACT BOX 103**

Blue toe syndrome secondary to showers of micro-emboli to digits distally can occur secondary to catheterization or angiography.

---

### Treatment

- Heparinization (100 units/kg loading dose, 10 units/kg/h for PTT 50–60).
- Hydration and alkalization of the urine. Urine output is maintained at >100cc/h. Myoglobinuria secondary to tissue ischemia can result in ATN.

*Revascularization* procedures within 6 hours of symptom onset to minimize morbidity.

- Embolectomy exposes the artery and uses a balloon-tip catheter that is passed distal to the embolus. The balloon is then blown up and removed to bring the embolus back with it.
- Bypass procedure.

# 41

# Mesenteric Vascular Disease

**Chronic Mesenteric Ischemia**

Chronic mesenteric ischemia is a progressive stenosis or occlusion of one or more of the supplying vessels (celiac, SMA, IMA). For symptoms to occur usually 2–3 of the vessels are occluded owing to the rich collateral circulation of the mesenteric bed.

*Symptoms*

Chronic mesenteric ischemia presents as
  • Abdominal pain following eating (food fear)
  • Weight loss
  • Epigastric bruit

*Diagnosis*

  • Duplex scanning
  • Arteriography

*Treatment*

  • Bypass or endarterectomy of the affected vessel

## Acute Mesenteric Ischemia

Acute mesenteric ischemia has an 80% mortality rate and is therefore treated as a surgical emergency. Embolization to the SMA is most common and usually originates from a cardiac source.

### Symptoms

Patients present with
- *Severe pain out of proportion to physical exam* without peritoneal signs
- Hyperdefecation, gut emptying
- Atrial fibrillation

Past medical history may also identify patients using digoxin, which is a potent splanchnic vasoconstrictor.

---

**FACT BOX 104**

Pain out of proportion to physical exam is the most common presentation for mesenteric ischemia.

---

### Diagnosis

- High index of suspicion and arteriogram

### Treatment

- Embolectomy or vasculature reconstruction.
- Following repair the bowel is assessed for viability. Necrotic bowel is resected while marginally viable bowel is left for a second-look operation to re-assess viability.

If *nonocclusive ischemia* is identified on arteriogram then
- Hydrate to optimize cardiac function.
- Vasodilating drugs.
- Repeat angiogram in 24 hours to re-assess.

**Renal Vasculature**

The most common cause of renal artery stenosis is arteriosclerosis or fibromuscular dysplasia.

### *Symptoms and Signs*

- Hypertension refractory to medical management

### *Diagnosis*

- Renal renin ratio >1.5 indicates stenosis.
- Renal systemic renin index.

### *Treatment*

- Pericutaneous dilatation (best with fibromuscular dysplasia)
- Renal artery endarterectomy
- Bypass to distal renal artery segment

# 42

# Carotid Artery Disease

**Statistics**

35% of carotid bruits have hemodynamically significant disease of and most predictive of MI.

>70% stenosis and symptomatic
- 9% two-year incidence of stroke (endarterectomy + ASA)
- 26% two-year incidence of stroke (ASA alone)

>60% stenosis and asymptomatic
- 5% five-year incidence of stroke to endarterectomy (with M&M <3%)
- 11% five-year incidence of stroke with no treatment

25% mortality from strokes (150K deaths annually)
85% result from embolization
Most occur at the carotid bifurcation.

**Anatomy**

External carotid artery branches:
- Superior thyroid
- Ascending pharyngeal
- Lingual
- Facial
- Occipital
- Posterior auricular

- Maxillary
- Superficial temporal

**Symptoms**

Transient Ischemic Attack (TIA)
- Focal episodes or neurologic symptoms of <5 minutes
- Resolution within 15 minutes without residual deficits
- Focal motor or sensory defect contralateral to involved artery
- Monocular blindness (amaurosis fugax) embolus to retinal vessel

Reversible Ischemic Neurologic Attack (RIND)—<48 hours
Stroke—irreversible changes

Carotid bruits are not reliable indicators of significant carotid vessel disease.
- 35% with bruits have hemodynamically significant disease.
- 50% of patients with hemodynamically significant disease will have bruits.
- Bruits are most predictive of coronary artery disease and the potential for myocardial infarction.

**Treatment**

Carotid endarterectomy (CEA) is the removal of the intima and sclerotic plaque from the artery. The artery is clamped or shunted. A back pressure >50 mm Hg is usually adequate for perfusion. Many surgeons prefer to shunt all CEAs.

**Complications**

*Wound Hematoma*—this may compromise the airway and should be evacuated at the bedside and explored as needed.
*Stroke*—rate should be 1%–4%.
*Hemodynamic*—the nerve to the carotid body may be sacrificed, interfering with baroreceptor mechanisms and producing blood pressure lability. Blood pressure should be monitored very closely.

**Nerve Damage**

- Recurrent laryngeal—hoarseness
- Hypoglossal—tongue deviation
- Superior laryngeal—weak voice

# 43

# Abdominal Aortic Aneurysm

## Statistics

- <4.5 cm 9% risk of rupture
- >7 cm 75% risk of rupture
- Expands 0.4 mm/yr
- 90% mortality with rupture

## Anatomy

- Aorta bifurcated at the level of the umbilicus
- 95% are infrarenal

## History

Severe central abdominal or back pain if ruptured. Occasionally the pain localizes to the lower abdomen, groin, or testis.

### Classic Triad of Rupture

- Abdominal pain
- Pulsatile abdominal mass
- Hypotension

FACT BOX **105**

Go to the OR immediately if:
- Abdominal pain
- Pulsatile abdominal mass
- Hypotension

## Differential Diagnosis

- Acute pancreatitis
- Dissecting aneurysm
- Mesenteric ischemia
- MI
- Perforated ulcer
- Diverticulosis

## Risk Factors for Rupture

- Recent rapid expansion
- Diameter >6 cm
- Hypertension

## Physical Exam

- Abdominal pulsation in 70% of patients. Signs of shock if ruptured.

## Labs

- Hemoglobin, hematocrit (or CBC with differential)
- Type and cross
- Coagulation studies (PT/PTT)

## Radiology

- *ABX* show calcifications in 60%–70%.
- *Ultrasound* is the method of choice and provides information about the diameter of the lumen.

- *CT with contrast* is usually performed prior to surgery to delineate the lumen and the thrombus and to check for venous anomalies and horseshoe kidney.
- *Aortography* is controversial. On the positive side it identifies the extent of involvement including the renal vasculature and demonstrated aortic outflow and the presence of occlusive disease, which would influence whether the graft extends to the common femoral artery.

---

**FACT BOX 106**

Angiogram does have an associated 1% mortality.

---

**Treatment**

*Elective Repair*

- >5 cm less than 20%–25% risk of eventual rupture.
- >6 cm have 45% risk of eventual rupture (should be repaired).
- Aneurysm >5 cm can be watched with follow-up ultrasound every 6 months. A normal aneurysm shows growth of ~0.5 cm in diameter per year. If there is growth of >0.5 cm in 3 months, rupture is more likely.

For all patients who are symptomatic, approximately 30% die in 1 month and 75% are dead in 6 months without treatment. In other words symptomatic aneurysm should be repaired regardless of size.

*Risk of No Treatment*

- Rupture
- Distal embolization
- Sudden aortic thrombosis
- Infection
- Aortointestinal fistula
- Aortic vena cava fistula

### Postoperative Complications Include

- Renal failure (4%–7%).
- Paraplegia from spinal cord ischemia (0.25%).
- Infected graft (1%–2%).
- Aortoenteric fistula secondary to infection. Aortoenteric fistula may present as minor herald GI bleed followed by exsanguination and usually involves the duodenum.
- Ischemic colitis from the ligation of the IMA, which presents as heme-positive diarrhea.

The most common associated problem is that of myocardial ischemia and insufficiency usually due to associated atherosclerotic lesions.

### Prognosis

- Mortality of elective operation is <5% but can be as high as 20% in high-risk patients.
- The 5-year survival after repair is 50%–75% with most common cause of death MI.
- Emergency repair for rupture is initial therapy including resuscitation from shock and invasive hemodynamic monitoring with emergent surgery. Mortality after rupture is 50% (if you include those that don't make it to the hospital it is 90%).

### Vascular Surgery—Most Commons and Facts

- Most common cause of mortality following vascular surgery is MI.
- Most common organism in infrarenal aorta is *Salmonella*.
- Most common graft infection is *Staph*.
- Splenic artery aneurysms rupture in 90% of pregnant patients.
- Popliteal is most common peripheral aneurysm; 50% are bilateral and 25% have associated AAA.
- Atherosclerosis occurs most commonly at proximal internal carotid, infrarenal aortic and superficial femoral arteries.

# 44

# Pediatric Surgery

## Duodenal Atresia

### Etiology

The pathogenesis is due to failure of recanalization of the gut lumen.

### Associated Anomalies

- Down syndrome (30%)
- Congenital heart defects (17%)
- Esophageal atresia (7%)
- Renal abnormalities (5%)

### Symptoms and Signs

- Often associated with polyhydramnios
- Vomiting soon after birth (bilious)
- Severe dehydration
- Failure to pass meconium

### Radiology

- Abdominal films identify a *double bubble*
- Diagnosis confirmed by upper GI series

### Management

- Laparotomy with duodenostomy or duodenojejunostomy

## Annular Pancreas

Most common form of external compression of second part of duodenum.

### Etiology

- Ring of pancreatic tissue due to persistent ventral primordium of the pancreas (normally rotated around the duodenum to join the dorsal bud to become the head of the pancreas)

### Treatment

- Duodenostomy (no direct intervention of the pancreas)

## Malrotation

- Most common cause of duodenal obstruction
- Results in volvulus of the midgut in 50% of patients
- Clockwise rotation (relieved by counterclockwise rotation)

### Symptoms and Signs

Patients present in the newborn period with
- Bilious vomiting
- Abdominal distention
- Dehydration

### Radiology

- Upper GI.
- Pathognomonic finding is *absence of ligament of Treitz* with duodenum in corkscrew configuration to the right of the spine.
- Plain film may identify single bubble of air in the vicinity of the left upper quadrant if a midgut volvulus is present.

### Treatment

*Ladd Procedure*—Division of the abnormal intestinal bands, appendectomy, and organization of the small gut on the right side of the peritoneal cavity and large bowel on the left side.

## Intestinal Obstruction

### General Symptoms and Signs

- Bilious vomiting
- Polyhydramnios with high atresia but not with more distal atresia
- Dehydrated
- Distention
- Failure to pass meconium

*Jejunoileal Atresia*—In utero vascular accident. Four types based on type of congenital defect. Plain films show markedly dilated loops of bowel. Contrast study identifies "micro" or "unused" colon. Management with laparotomy excision of the atretic segment and primary anastomosis of the bowel (usually end to side).

### Meconium Ileus

Associated with cystic fibrosis (AR incidence of 1 in 20 carriers) can lead to perforation, cystic dilatation. Abdomen films may show distended gas-filled loops of bowel, soap-bubble appearance of distal ileum, and possible calcifications.

*Treatment*—Small concretions of distal ileum can be irrigated with evacuation of meconium, excision of atretic segments or dilatation and creation of ileostomy.

- Sweat test should be performed to identify possible cystic fibrosis.

### Hirschprung's Disease

Complete colonic obstruction due to absence of ganglion cells in the distal gut.

### Symptoms

Most are diagnosed in infancy with failure to pass meconium within 24 hours after birth. May be associated with vomiting and abdominal distention. If undiagnosed early, may lead to severe constipation, entercolitis, dehydration, and sepsis.

*BE*

- Distal bowel (aganglionic segment) in spasm and proximal bowel (normal) dilated due to pseudo-obstruction.

*Biopsy*

- Rectal biopsy will fail to identify ganglion cells in submucosal or intramuscular nerve plexus.

*Treatment*

Exploration in newborn period with biopsy and diversion proximal to transition zone. Definitive procedure is done at the age of 1 with weight of 20–25 lbs.

- *Swenson's Procedure*—resection of aganglionic intestine and two-layer anastomosis of pulled-through normal bowel to the rectum.
- *Duhamel's Procedure*—50% of circumference of the most distal bowel segment is ganglionic and 50% aganglionic. The innervated bowel is brought behind the preserved rectum and sutured together and stapled to form a common chamber. The remaining aganglionic bowel is left.
- *Soave's Procedure*—a mucosectomy of the most distal aspect of the aganglionic bowel is done and normal bowel pulled through this seromuscular sleeve and anastomosed at the anal verge.

## Omphalocele

Defect of the umbilical ring with extruded abdominal contents covered by sac (peritoneum and amnion).

### *Statistics*

- 1 in 1000
- 50% associated with other GI, C, GU, MS, CNS, and chromosomal abnormalities.

### Treatment

- Decompress bowel with NG tube
- IVF
- Prophylactic antibiotics

### Surgery

- Primary closure of abdominal wall.
- Use silo to house abdominal contents and decrease size over 4–7 days.
- Betadine spray or silvadene over defect to form eschar with subsequent epithelialization. Repair can then be accomplished at a later time.

## Gastroschisis

Defect in abdominal wall lateral to umbilicus *not* covered by a sac
Usually not associated with other abnormalities and relatively uncommon

### Treatment

- NG tube
- IVF
- Antibiotics

### Surgery

Reduction of viscera and abdominal closure (may require use of SILO)

## Esophageal Atresia and Fistula

Atresia is blind-ending pouch without fistula.

### Statistics

- 50% with associated anomalies (VACTERL)
- 85% TE fistulae are type C

## Symptoms

- Excessive secretions and poor feeding

## Diagnosis

- NG tube cannot be passed effectively with coiling of tube.

## Treatment

- NG suction and gastrostomy for feeding and/or drainage

## Surgery

- Stretching of blind pouch to re-anastomose to stomach

## TE Fistula

*Type A*—esophageal atresia without fistula (8%)
*Type B*—proximal TE fistula (<1%)
*Type C*—proximal esophageal atresia with distal TE fistula (most common, 85%)
*Type D*—proximal atresia with proximal and distal TE fistula
*Type E*—H type TE fistula without atresia

## Signs and Symptoms

- Excessive secretions
- Respiratory compromise
- Postprandial regurgitation

## Treatment

- Surgical re-anastomosis and closure of fistula

## Diaphragmatic Hernia

Defect in diaphragm allows abdominal viscera into thorax.

## Statistics

- 90% left side posterior lateral

## Types

*Bochdalek*—posterolateral to left
*Morgagni*—anterior parasternal

## Diagnosis

- Intrauterine
- Respiratory distress from lung hypoplasia

## Treatment

- Primary repair of defect when discovered
- Survival dependent on degree of pulmonary hypoplasia

### Necrotizing Enterocolitis

## Etiology

- Disease of bowel wall leading to bacterial invasion
- Pneumatosis intestinalis
- Affects premature infants that have been fed and is more common in infants with complicated perinatal course

## Signs and Symptoms

- Sepsis
- Acidosis
- Respiratory compromise
- Abdominal distention
- Bloody stools

## Radiology

- Pneumatosis intestinalis
- Distended loops
- Portal venous gas
- Free air

## Labs

- Decreasing Hgb and platelets

243

## Treatment

- Primarily medical with surgical intervention for complications such as perforation

## Surgery

- Ischemic bowel is resected with diversion
- Marginal bowel is left for second-look operation 24 hours later
- Complications may include development of strictures and progressive intestinal obstruction

## Umbilical Hernia

Fascial wall defect more common in black than white infants

## Treatment

- Small (<2 cm) will close on their own and usually do not require repair (by 2 years)
- >2 cm will require surgical repair (3–4 years of age)

## Intussusception

Telescoping of bowel into another portion of bowel
10 months to 2 years old

## Signs and Symptoms

- Irritability
- Fever
- Waxing and waning pain
- Currant jelly stool (blood and mucus)
- Dance sign—palpable mass in right upper quadrant with empty right lower quadrant

## Treatment

IVF to correct dehydration
<24 hours can usually be corrected with contrast enema

## Undescended Testes

- 1% of general population.
- A testis that cannot be palpated or manipulated into the scrotum.
- Often associated with inguinal hernia.
- If undescended at birth it should reach scrotum by 2–3 months of age.

### Treatment

- Surgical correction before the age of 2.
- Patients >2 yr have increased incidence of dysplasia and subsequent malignancy ($9 \times$).
- Surgery does not eliminate risk of CA but places the testis in location where it can be examined.

## Neuroblastoma

- Neural crest origin
- 75% in abdomen from adrenals
- 90% secrete catecholamines
- Most common abdominal neoplasm in children

### Diagnosis

- Palpable abdominal mass
- Likely crosses midline

### Symptoms and Signs

- Hypertension
- Tachycardia
- Sweat and pallor
- Diarrhea and vomiting
- Anemia, fever, and malaise
- Horner's syndrome

### Radiology

- KUB
- Bone scan
- IVP
- CT with contrast

### Treatment

*Stage I and II*—surgery and chemotherapy
*Stage II with nodes or positive tumor markers*—surgery, radiation, chemotherapy
*Stage III and IV*—multimodal chemotherapy, surgery, total body irradiation, BMT

### Survival

- Stage I    100%
- Stage II    80%
- Stage III    40%
- Stage IV    10%

# 45

# Molecular Surgery

*Molecular surgery* is the identification and manipulation of molecular and genetic factors in surgery-related disease. The result of such manipulation is reduction in tumor size, regression of metastatic disease, adjuvant therapy, immune enhancement, rapid recovery from surgical procedures, etc.

### Genetic Components

*DNA (deoxyribonucleic acid):* DNA is a double-stranded molecule consisting of the four DNA nucleotides: adenine (A), guanine (G), cytosine (C), and thymine (T). Base pairs form only between A and T and between G and C; thus the base sequence of each single strand can be deduced from that of its partner.

*Ribonucleic acid (RNA):* Found in the nucleus and cytoplasm of cells; involved in protein synthesis and other chemical activities of the cell. Classes of RNA molecules include messenger RNA (mRNA), transfer RNA (tRNA), ribosomal RNA (rRNA), and other RNAs, each serving a different purpose.

  • *Introns:* The DNA base sequences interrupting the protein-coding sequences of a gene; these sequences are transcribed into RNA but are cut out of the message before it is translated into protein. Possibly representing evolutionary and developmental genes.

  • *Exons:* The protein-coding DNA sequences of a gene.

*Ribosomes:* Small cellular components composed of specialized rRNA and protein; site of protein synthesis.

*Messenger RNA (mRNA):* RNA that serves as a template for protein synthesis.

*Transfer RNA (tRNA):* A class of RNA having structures with triplet nucleotide sequences that are complementary to the triplet nucleotide coding sequences of mRNA. The role of tRNAs in protein synthesis is to bond with amino acids and transfer them to the ribosomes, where proteins are assembled according to the genetic code carried by mRNA.

### Enzymes

*Endonuclease:* An enzyme that cleaves its nucleic acid substrate at internal sites in the nucleotide sequence.

*Exonuclease:* An enzyme that cleaves nucleotides sequentially from free ends of a linear nucleic acid substrate.

### Gene Therapy (Molecular Surgery)

Gene therapy is the introduction of genetic material into cells for the purpose of repairing, replacing or attenuating function. Gene therapy has progressed to providing new genetic machinery to cells to help them fight disease of neoplastic processes. This unique form of therapy targets genetic material with the use of viral and retroviral vectors as a delivery vehicle. The cell may be triggered to release the product of the new gene, which can act locally on neighboring cells or enter the circulation for delivery to distant cells (i.e., endocrine or paracrine function).

*Vector:* A genetic tool used to transmit genetic information and insert it into the genome.

*Bacteriophage or phage:* A virus whose natural host is a bacterial cell. Used to transfect genetic material into bacteria.

*Plasmid:* Autonomously replicating, extrachromosomal circular DNA molecules, distinct from the normal bacterial genome and nonessential for cell survival under nonselective conditions. Some plasmids are capable of integrating into the host genome. A number of artificially constructed plasmids are used as cloning vectors. Associated with antibiotic resistance.

*Cosmid:* Artificially constructed cloning vector containing the cos gene of phage lambda. Cosmids can be packaged in lambda phage particles for infection into *E. coli*; this permits cloning of larger DNA fragments (up to 45 kb) that can be introduced into bacterial hosts in plasmid vectors.

*Yeast artificial chromosome (YAC):* A vector used to clone DNA fragments (up to 400 kb); it is constructed from the telomeric, centromeric, and replication origin sequences needed for replication in yeast cells. Compare cloning vector, cosmid.

*Retroviruses:* These are generally used for ex vivo gene delivery, i.e., the injection of cells that were genetically engineered by infection outside the body, rather than by in vivo infection with the retrovirus itself. Useful in that it integrates into the host genome.

*Adenoviruses:* These readily infect nondividing cells, can be produced in large numbers, infect adult tissues, and remain extra-chromosomal. Limitations of adenoviruses are that they infect all tissues (including the germ line), adenoviral vectors are immunogenic, reducing the length of time available for the expression of the gene, and making repeated administration of the vector impossible.

*Antisense Technology:* These short oligonucleotide sequences are introduced into cells and subsequently form DNA triplex at its complementary region. This results in an inhibition of transcription at this site, decreasing expression of the gene.

*Liposomes:* These combine readily with cell membranes and are being used to deliver genes, sometimes as aerosols. Liposomes are also being tested in conjunction with viruses to enhance localized delivery of genes.

**Genetic Disorders**

*Mutation:* Any heritable change in DNA sequence.

*Oncogene:* A gene, one or more forms of which are associated with cancer. Many oncogenes are involved, directly or indirectly, in controlling the rate of cell growth.

*Tumor Suppressor Gene:* A gene that functions to suppress cell division and growth. Must lose both copies to lose function.

*Polygenic Disorders:* Genetic disorders resulting from the combined action of alleles of more than one gene (e.g., heart disease, diabetes, and some cancers). Although such disorders are inherited, they depend on the simultaneous presence of several alleles; thus the hereditary patterns are usually more complex than those of single-gene disorders.

*Single-Gene Disorder:* Hereditary disorder caused by a mutant allele of a single gene (e.g., Duchenne muscular dystrophy, retinoblastoma, sickle cell disease).

Potential targets for molecular surgery include:
- Enhancing the host immune recognition of tumor cells. Use of cytokine and interleukin delivery
- Inducing apoptosis in tumor cells
- Delivery of tumor suppressor genes

## Breast Cancer

Less than 5% of breast cancers are familial. Associated genes are:
- *BRCA*-1
- *BRCA*-2
- *HER*-2/*neu*

## Colon Cancer

Progression of colorectal carcinoma from adenoma to cancer through mutations of a series of genes.
- ras
- Chromosome 5q—APC (adenomatous polyposis coli)
- Chromosome 17p—p53
- Chromosome 18q—DCC (deleted in colorectal carcinoma)
- Chromosome 2p—hMSH2
- Chromosome 3—hMSH1

### *Oncogenes*

| TABLE 45.1 Oncogenes in Cancer | |
|---|---|
| c-myc | Breast and lung cancer |
| n-myc | Neuroblastoma |
| l-myc | Lung cancer |
| Erb B-2 | Breast and ovarian cancer |
| K-ras | Pancreatic and colon cancers |

## Suppresser Genes

**TABLE 45.2**
**Tumor Suppressor Genes**

| | |
|---|---|
| *p53* | Many (50% of genetic cancers) |
| *Rb1* | Retinoblastoma, small cell lung cancer |
| *WT1* | Lung cancer |
| *APC* | Familial polyposis coli |
| *DCC* | Colon cancer |

**TABLE 45.3**
**Oncogene Functions**

| *Oncogene* | Function |
|---|---|
| *erb B* | Part of EGF receptor |
| *Her-2/neu (c-erb B2)* | Associated with protein tyrosine kinase |
| *src* | Tyrosine kinase |
| *RET* | Tyrosine kinase |
| *ras* | GTP binding/GTPase |
| *myc* | Transcription factor |
| *fos* | Cell cycle transcription factor |
| *jun* | Cell cycle transcription factor |
| *bcl-1* | Activates cell cycle kinases |
| *bcl-2* | Antagonizes programmed cell death |

## Apoptosis

Apoptosis, or programmed cell death, is a rapidly growing field in medical research.

- Genetically encoded program to produce cell death and maintain homeostasis
- Involved in human development, cellular differentiation, normal cell turnover
- In many cancers this mechanism is turned off, leading to unregulated proliferation
- Complex pathways associated with the apoptotic process
- Receptors CD95, FasL, TNF

## Apoptotic Signals

- Caspsases (caspsase 8 primary end event)
- Tumor suppressors (p53)

- p21, p16, p14
- Bak, Bax, E2F-1
- Chemotherapeutic agents (alkalating)

### *Anti-Apoptotic*

- Bcl-2
- Mutations in suppressors, oncogenes

## Immunology

### *Cytokines*

*IL-1*

- Causes fever
- Stimulates release of TNF-$\alpha$ IL-6, IL-8, platelet-activating factor, prostaglandins
- Stimulates T and B cells
- Promotes acute-phase protein production
- Increases endothelial procoagulant activity

*IL-2*

- Stimulates release of TNF-$\alpha$ and IFN-$\gamma$
- Causes hypotension
- Enhances T-cell proliferation and cytotoxic T-cell function

*IL-6*

- Enhances neutrophil activation
- Promotes T- and B-cell activation
- Stimulates acute-phase protein production
- Fever

*IL-12*

- Promotes Th1-cell differentiation

*TNF-α*

- Stimulates release of IL-1, IL-6, platelet-activating factor, prostaglandins
- Promotes activation of neutrophils, monocytes
- Increases expression of adhesion molecules
- Activates complement and coagulation cascades
- Increases vascular permeability
- Hypotension
- Fever

*IFN-γ*

- Stimulates release of TNF-α, IL-1, IL-6
- Promotes macrophage activation

### Tumor Markers

**TABLE 45.4**
**Tumor Markers**

| Marker | Tumor Type |
| --- | --- |
| Carcinoembryonic antigen (CEA) | Colorectal, pancreatic, breast, lung |
| Alpha-fetoprotein (AFP) | Hepatocellular carcinomas, testicular cancers |
| Beta-human chorionic gonado-tropin (βHCG) | Testicular tumors, tropho-blastic, gestational tumors |
| Prostate-specific antigen (PSA) | Prostate cancer |
| CA 15–3 | Breast cancer |
| CA 19–9, CA 50, CA 242 | Pancreatic, colorectal, gastric |
| CA 125 | Ovarian, other gynecologic tumors |
| Neuron-specific enolase (NSE) | Neuroendocrine tumors, medullary thyroid cancer, small cell lung cancer, islet cell tumors, carcinoids |
| erb B-2 | Breast, ovarian, stomach |

# 46

# Basic Biostatistics

Basic biostatistics are necessary for the understanding and evaluation of current research and publication. Basic biostatistics are also a part of every Shelf Surgery Board Exam.

*Mean.* Average of values.

*Median.* The value in the middle of a data set.

*Mode.* Most common value in a population set.

*Standard Deviation.* A value given to identify how much variation there exists around the mean.

- One STD, 68% of the population falls in this range.
- Two STD, 95% of the population falls in this range.

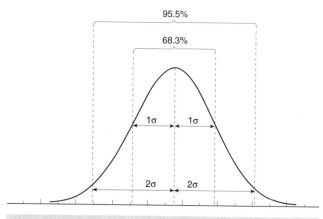

**FIGURE 46.1**
Normal distribution. σ = Standard Deviation

*Standard Error of the Mean.* Is similar to the STD but it compensates for the sample size in a study. It is equal to the STD divided by the square root of *n*.

*Incidence.* Incidence is the number of new individuals developing a disease in a given period of time (e.g., 1 year) divided by the number of individuals at risk during that same time.

*Prevalence.* The number of individuals in a population that have the disease.

## Research Studies

*Prospective Studies.* Prospective or cohort studies begin by identifying a specific population (cohorts) that are free of the disease at the start of the study and subsequently assess exposure to the risk factor of interest.

• A prospective, randomized, controlled study is the definitive evaluation of a particular treatment.

*Retrospective Studies.* Case-control studies are subjects with disease (case) and those without (control) and information about prior risk factors is evaluated. These are typically chart review reports and are compared with odds ratio.

*Cross-Sectional Studies.* Provide information at one point in time.

## Bias

When evaluating a paper in the literature, it is important to determine if any bias exists that may skew the significance of the report. Examples are:

*Selection Bias*—subjects are assigned to groups that differ with regard to outside factors not involved in the study. For example, when testing a drug for decreasing the risk of MI the investigator inadvertently places people who exercise in the treatment arm and people who do not in the placebo arm.

*Lead-Time Bias*—identifying people with disease at an earlier point in the disease process. This artificially leads to increased survival.

*Recall Bias*—inaccurate patient recall of the degree of exposure of the risk factor. This is the limitation in a retrospective study.

*Confounding*—is the inability to determine which variable is producing the effect. For example, if testing a new drug that decreases risk of CAD in a patient who also exercises and drinks one glass of wine a day, it may be difficult to determine what is causing the reduction in risk.

**Risk Analysis**

### TABLE 46.1
### Two-Way Table

|  | True + (Disease) | True – (No Disease) | Total |
|---|---|---|---|
| Risk Factor + | a | c | a + c |
| Risk Factor – | b | d | b + d |
| Total | a + b | c + d | Total N |

*Relative Risk* is the ratio of individuals with disease and risk factor to individuals with disease and no risk factor. Used in prospective studies.

$$RR = \frac{\frac{a}{a+c}}{\frac{b}{b+d}}$$

*Odds Ratio* is an estimate of the relative risk when incidence data is not available. It is equal to the relative risk divided by the ratio of persons without risk with disease to persons without risk without disease. Used in retrospective studies.

$$OR = \frac{ad}{bc}$$

**Testing**

*Sensitivity* is the ability of a test to detect people with disease (true +).

*Specificity* is the ability of a test to detect people without disease (true –).

*Positive Predictive Value* detects the probability of having a positive test for individuals with disease.

*Sensitivity*

$$\frac{true+}{(true+)+(false-)}$$

*Specificity*

$$\frac{true-}{(true-)+(false+)}$$

*False Negative Rate*

$$\frac{false-}{(false-)+(true+)}$$

## Statistical Analysis

*Hypothesis* states that there is a difference between tested groups.

*Null Hypothesis* states that there is no difference between tested groups.

*Type I Error* occurs when the null hypothesis is rejected when it is actually true.

*Type II Error* ($\beta$) occurs when the null hypothesis is not rejected although it is false.

*Power* is the probability that a test will reach a particular conclusion. Defined by:

$$Power(\alpha) = 1 - \beta$$

In other words, the power determines how many patients are needed to identify a difference (accept the hypothesis and reject the null hypothesis).

*Probability* (p) represents the chance of a type I error. If a *p* value is equal to or less than .05, it is unlikely that a type I error has been made.

## Tests of Significance

Various tests are available to determine the "*p* value" and therefore determine if the differences between two or more groups are real or by chance.

### t-test

Unpaired used to test two means taken at time *x*.

Paired used for two means taken at time *x* and time *y* (before treatment and after treatment).

257

## ANOVA (Analysis of Variance)

This test is used if comparing more than two groups.
One-way used for >2 groups with one variable being tested.
Two-way used for >2 groups with two variables being tested.

## $\chi^2$

Tests frequencies (rates) between two groups to determine if there
is a statistical difference.

### Multiple Regression

Tests the relationship between variables in a given sample controlling for identified variables. This can be used to determine if there
is a correlation between several variables and the disease. For
example, you can determine if age, weight, smoking history, and
exercise correlate with coronary artery disease.

# 47

# Procedures

## Central Line Placement

### General

1. Check PT/PTT for possible coagulopathy.
2. Place rolled towel between the shoulder blades and place in Trendelenburg for better exposure of the vessels.
3. Gown, glove.
4. Sterility prep and drape the area (chlorohexadine or Betadine).
5. Infiltrate the site with 1%–2% lidocaine using a 25-G needle aspirating as you proceed. Anesthetize the clavicular edge.
6. Using 18-G needle insert slowly to identify the vein.
7. When blood returns stabilize the needle and remove the syringe, placing a finger over the exposed needle to prevent embolism.
8. Place guide wire through the needle and advance. Withdraw the needle, holding on to the wire at all times.
9. Nick the skin with #11 scalpel blade, insert dilator over the wire, and then withdraw the dilator.
10. Advance the catheter over the wire (18 cm for left SCV and IJ, 15 cm for right SCV, 12 cm for right IJ).
11. Remove wire, check for free return of blood, and flush with NS.

12. Suture to skin and place occlusive dressing (Tegaderm with 2 × 2 gauze) over site.
13. Order STAT CXR to check placement before use. The catheter tip should be at SVC atrial junction.

*Internal Jugular Central Approach*

Locate triangle formed between the two heads of the SCM muscle. This can be done by placing your index finger in the sternal notch and middle finger on the clavicle. Insert the needle at the apex of the triangle with a 45-degree angle and aim needle toward the ipsilateral nipple. The vein is not very deep at this location.

*Internal Jugular Posterior Approach*

Identify area three fingerbreadths above the clavicle. Insert the needle under the SCM at this point aiming anterially to the suprasternal notch.

*Subclavian Vein Infraclavicular*

Insert needle 1–2 cm below the junction of the medial and middle thirds of the clavicle. Advance the needle parallel to the chest wall aiming 1 cm above the suprasternal notch. When the clavicle is reached push the needle under the clavicle with your left index finger.

**Pulmonary Artery Catheter**

1. Cannulate central vein using Seldinger technique as described. Introduce the catheter sheath (Cordis) and suture in place with confirmation of adequate blood return.
2. Attach IV tubing to the Cordis line.
3. Check Swan-Ganz catheter to ensure that it is functioning correctly. Check balloon with 1.5 cc air, flush lumens with saline/heparin solution, and eliminate bubbles.
4. Gently shake catheter tip to confirm pressure changes.
5. Insert catheter slowly until CVP is encountered (15–20 cm).
6. Inflate balloon and advance into right atrium and then right ventricle. Advance the catheter smoothly and quickly into the pulmonary artery.

7. Advance into PCW position and deflate the balloon. If pulmonary artery wave form returns you have a good position. If wedge pressure remains you need to withdraw and recheck. (Always deflate the balloon before withdrawing.)

## Chest Tube Placement

1. Abduct arm on side of pneumothorax and place behind head.
2. Identify site for tube placement midaxillary line to anterior axillary line at the fourth intercostal space.
3. Widely prep the area and drape in sterile fashion.
4. Identify the fourth or fifth rib and infiltrate the area with 1% lidocaine (10–20 mL). Go down to rib and over it superiorly. Liberal use of lidocaine will help attenuate the pain with placement.
5. Make 1- to 2-cm incision over the rib.
6. Using Kelly clamp, bluntly dissect a short (1–2 rib) subcutaneous tunnel over the superior portion of the rib.
7. Once entering the pleural space insert a finger to confirm intrapleural location and check for adhesions.
8. Insert the chest tube (28–36 F) by clamping the end with the Kelly and advancing it into the chest. Clamp the distal end of the tube as a hemothorax will quickly evacuate if the end is left open.
9. Direct it superiorly for pneumothorax or inferiorly for effusion.
10. Suture tube to skin using 0 Ethibond.
11. Dress with $4 \times 4$s and silk tape.

# 48

# Surgical Medications

**Pain Meds**

meperidine (Demerol) 25–50 mg IV/IM/PO q3–4h
morphine sulfate (0.1–0.2 mg/kg) 2–4 mg IV/IM q2–3h
oxycodone (Oxycontin) 30–60 mg PO q12h
hydrocodone/acetaminophen (500) (Lortab) (2.5/5/7.5/10) 1–2
 PO q4–6h
oxycodone/acetaminophen (325) (Percocet) (5/7.5/10) 1–2 PO
 q4–6h
oxycodone/acetaminophen (325) per 5 mL (Roxicet) (5/7.5/10)
 5–10 mL q4–6h
oxycodone/ASA 325 (Percodan) (5) 1–2 PO q4–6h
propoxyphene/acetaminophen (Darvocet) (50–100/650) N-50,
 N-100 1–2 PO q4–6h prn
hydrocodone/ibuprofen (Vicoprofen) (7.5/200) 1–2 PO q6h
Tylenol #3 1–2 PO q3–4h
ketorolac (Toradl) 30 mg IV/IM q6; 10 mg PO q4 (watch renal
 function)
tramadol (Ultram) 50–100 mg PO q4–6h

**Anesthesia/Sedatives**

lorazepam (Ativan) 1–2 mg IV/PO q6h
midazolam (Versed) 1 mg IV titrate to effect
propofol (Diprovan) 1–3 mg/kg IV (10 mg/mL)
etomidate (Amidate) 0.2–0.5 mg/kg IV (2 mg/mL)

thiopental sodium (Pentothal) 4–6 mg/kg IV (25 mg/mL)
succinylcholine (Anectine) 1 mg/kg IV (20 mg/mL)
vecuronium (Norcuron) 0.1 mg/kg IV

**Reversal Agents**

flumazenil (Romazicon) 0.2 mg IV, then 0.2 mg/min to effect or
    1 mg
naloxone (Narcan) 0.01 mg/kg, 0.4–2 mg IV/IM/SC/ET

**Antibiotics**

*First-Generation Cephalosporin*

cefazolin (Ancef, Kefzol) 1 g IV
cephalexin (Keflex) 250–500 mg PO qid

*Second-Generation Cephalosporin*

cefoxitin 1–2 g IV/IM q6–8h
cefotetan (Cefotan) 2 g IV q12 × 48h

*Third-Generation Cephalosporin*

ceftazidime (Fortaz) 1–2 g IV q8–12h
ceftriaxone (Rocephin) 1–2 g IV/IM q24h
cefotaxime (Claforan) 1–2 g IV/IM q6–8h

*Penicillins*

amoxil 250–500 mg PO tid
amoxicillin clavulanate (Augmentin) 250–500 mg tid
ampicillin 1–2 g IV/IM q4–6h
oxacillin 1–2 g IV/IM q4–6h
ampicillin sulbactam (Unasyn) 1.5–3 g IV q6h
piperacillin tazobactam (Zosyn) 3.375 g IV q6h
ticarcillin clavulanate (Timentin) 3.1 g IV q4–6h

*Aminoglycoside*

gentamicin 1 mg/kg IV/IM q8h

## *Macrolides*

erythromycin 250–500 mg PO bid

azithromycin (Zithromax) 500 mg PO day 1, then 250 mg PO
    qd to day 5

clarithromycin (Biaxin) 250–500 mg PO bid

## *Fluoroquinolones*

ciprofloxacin (Cipro) 200–400 mg IV q12h, 250–750 PO bid

levofloxacin (Levoquin) 500 mg IV qd

ofloxacin (Floxin) 200–400 mg IV/PO q12h

## *Other*

aztreonam (Azactam) 0.5–2 g IV/IM q6–12h

chloramphenicol (Chloromycetin) 50–100 mg/kg/d IV/PO
    divided q6h

clindamycin (Cleocin) 600–1200 mg IV divided q6–12h,
    150–450 mg PO qid

imipenem-cilastatin (Primaxin) 250–1000 mg IV/IM q6–8h

metronidazole (Flagyl) 250–750 mg PO tid (2 g single dose
    trich, BV)

vancomycin (Vancocin) 500 mg IV q6 over 1 hour, *C. difficile*
    40 mg/kg PO up to 2000 mg/d tid or qid

## Antihypertensives

propranolol (Inderal) 40 mg PO bid to 640 mg

labetalol (Trandate) 20 mg IV q6h prn up to 300 mg/d

metoprolol (Lopressor) 50 mg PO bid, 5 mg IV q5min to
    15 mg

esmolol (Brevibloc) 500 mcg/kg over 1 min, 50–200
    mcg/kg/min drip

hydralazine (Apresoline) 10–40 mg IV/IM q4–6h up to 300
    mg/d

benazepril (Lotensin) 10 mg po qd to 80 mg qd

enalapril (Vasotec) 1.25 mg IV q6h; 5 mg PO qd

nifedipine (Procardia) 10 mg PO tid; Procardia XL 30–60 mg
    PO qd

verapamil (Calan) SVT 5–10 mg IV over 2 min 80 mg tid
(Calan SR 120 qd)
diltaizem (Cardizem) a-fib 20-mg bolus with 10-mg/h drip

## Diuretics

chlorothiazide (Diuril) 250–500 mg IV/PO qd/bid
furosemide (Lasix) 20–80 mg IV/PO qd/bid
bumetanide (Bumex) 1–2 mg IV qd/bid
acetazolamide (Diamox) 250 mg IV/PO q8–24h
spironolactone (Aldactone) 50–100 mg PO qd

## GI

metoclopramide (Reglan) 10 mg IV q6h
promethazine (Phenergan) 12.5–25 mg PO/IM/PR
odansetron (Zofran) 4 mg IV over 2–5 minutes × 1
docusate sodium (Colace) 100 mg PO qd
famotidine (Pepcid) 20 mg IV q12h
ranitidine (Zantac) 300 qhs; 50 mg IV q6–8h

## *H. pylori* Treatment

lansoprazole (Prevacid) 30 mg PO bid + clarithromycin (Biaxin)
500 mg PO bid + amoxicillin 1 g PO bid × 14 days
omeprazole (Prilosec) 20 mg PO qd + clarithromycin (Biaxin)
500 mg PO bid + amoxicillin 1 g PO bid × 14 days

## Pulmonary

theophylline 100–300 mg PO tid/qid
albuterol 2 puffs q4–6h, 2–4 mg PO tid/qid
terbutaline 2 puffs q4–6h, 5 mg PO tid
metoproterenol 2–3 puffs q3–4h
triamcinolone (Azmacort) 2 puffs tid/qid
flunisolide (AeroBid) 2 puffs bid
ipratropium (Combivent) 2 puffs q4–6h prn

## Cardiac Medications in ICU

dobutamine 5–25 mcg/kg/min

amrinone (Inocor) 5–25 mcg/kg/min

dopamine renal dose <5 mcg/kg/min, pressor/ionotroph doses
    5–20 mcg/kg/min

phenylephrine 40–60 mcg/min

norepinephrine 2–4 mcg/min

nitroglycerin 5–20 mcg/min

nitroprusside 0.02–0.7 mcg/min

## Hematology

enoxaparin (Lovenox) 30 mg SQ bid for DVT prophylaxis

heparin 100 U/kg loading dose, then ~1000U/h drip

protamine 1 mg per 100 U heparin

clopidogrel (Plavix) 75 mg PO qd

pentoxifylline (Trental) 400 mg PO tid

cilostazol (Pletal) 100 mg PO bid

# 49

# Equations

## Fluids and Electrolytes

Anion Gap = $Na - (Cl + HCO_3)$
Serum Osmolality = $2Na + BUN/2.8 + Glu/18$
TBW = $0.6 \times$ (weight in kg)
$H_2O$ Deficit = $0.6$ (kg)(serum $Na - 140$)/140
Parkland Formula = $2 - 4$ mL $\times$ TBSA $\times$ wt in kg
Corrected Na = $(Glu - 100) \times 0.016$
Corrected Ca = $[(3.5 - albumin) \times 0.8] + Ca$

## Renal Equations

FeNa = $(U/P)_{Na}/(U/P)_{Cr}$

## Hemodynamic Equations

Cardiac Output (CO) = $HR \times SV$
$O_2$ Delivery ($DO_2$) = $CO \times CaO_2$
Arterial $O_2$ Content ($CaO_2$) = $1.36(Hgb)(SaO_2) + 0.003(PaO_2)$
A-a Gradient = $[(713 \times FiO_2) - pCO_2/0.8] - pO_2$

# 50

# Common Abbreviations

| | |
|---|---|
| A/O: | Alert and oriented |
| AAA: | Abdominal aortic aneurysm |
| ABC: | Airway, Breathing, Circulation |
| ABG: | Arterial blood gases |
| Abx: | Antibiotics |
| ac: | Latin "ante cibum"; before meals |
| ACE: | Angiotensin-converting enzyme |
| ACLS: | Advanced cardiac life support |
| ADH: | Antidiuretic hormone |
| Ad Lib: | As desired |
| AF: | Atrial fibrillation |
| AFB: | Acid-fast bacilli |
| AFP: | Alpha-fetoprotein |
| AKA: | Above the knee amputation |
| AMA: | Against medical advice |
| AMI: | Acute myocardial infarction |
| AOS: | Arrived on scene |
| AP: | Anterior-Posterior—x-ray view |
| APR: | Abdominoperineal resection |
| ARDS: | Adult respiratory distress syndrome |
| ARF: | Acute renal failure |
| ASA: | Acetylsalicylic acid (aspirin) |
| ASAP: | As soon as possible |
| ATN: | Acute tubular necrosis |

| | |
|---|---|
| AV: | Arteriovenous |
| AVM: | Arteriovenous malformation |
| AVPU: | Alert, Verbal, Pain, Unresponsive (trauma alertness scale) |
| | |
| B: | Bilateral |
| B1: | Billroth 1 |
| B2: | Billroth 2 |
| BAL: | Blood alcohol level |
| BE: | Base excess |
| bid: | Bis in die (twice daily) |
| BiPAP: | Bilevel positive airway pressure |
| BKA: | Below the knee amputation |
| BLS: | Basic life support |
| BM: | Bowel movement |
| BMI: | Body mass index |
| BP: | Blood pressure |
| BPH: | Benign prostatic hypertrophy |
| BRB: | Bright red blood |
| BRBPR: | Bright red blood per rectum |
| BS: | Bowel sounds, (+)BS (don't ever say "positive BS," say either present or not present) |
| BS: | Breath sounds |
| BSA: | Body surface area |
| BSO: | Bilateral salpingo-oophorectomy |
| BUN: | Blood urea nitrogen |
| Bx: | Biopsy |
| | |
| c̄: | cum (with) |
| c/c/e: | clubbing, cyanosis, edema of extremities |
| C&DB: | Cough & deep breathe |
| C&S: | Culture & sensitivity |
| c/o: | complains of |
| c/w: | consistent with |
| Ca: | Calcium |
| CA: | Cancer, Carcinoma |
| CABG: | Coronary arterial bypass graft |
| CAD: | Coronary artery disease |
| CBC: | Complete blood count |

| | |
|---|---|
| CBD: | Common bile duct |
| CC: | Chief complaint |
| CCU: | Coronary/Cardiac care unit |
| CEA: | Carcinoembryonic antigen |
| CHD: | Coronary heart disease, congenital heart disease |
| CHF: | Congestive heart failure |
| CHI: | Closed head injury |
| CHO: | carbohydrate |
| CI: | Cardiac index |
| CIS: | Carcinoma in situ |
| CK: | Creatine phosphokinase |
| ck: | Check |
| Cl: | Chloride |
| CME: | Continuing medical education |
| CMP: | Comprehensive metabolic panel |
| CMV: | Cytomegalovirus |
| CO: | Cardiac output; Carbon monoxide |
| $CO_2$: | Carbon dioxide |
| COPD: | Chronic obstructive pulmonary disease |
| CP: | Chest pain |
| CPAP: | Continuous positive airway pressure |
| CPR: | Cardiopulmonary resuscitation |
| CRF: | Chronic renal failure |
| C-scope: | Colonoscopy |
| CT: | CAT scan (computed axial tomography) |
| CTA: | Clear to auscultation |
| CTAB: | Clear to auscultation bilaterally |
| CVA: | Cerebrovascular accident |
| CVP: | Central venous pressure |
| CXR: | Chest x-ray |
| Cx: | Cultures |
| | |
| D/C: | Discharge, Discontinue, or Disconnect |
| D5/LR: | 5% dextrose in lactated Ringer's |
| D50: | Dextrose 50% |
| D5W: | Dextrose 5% in water |
| DBP: | Diastolic blood pressure |
| DCIS: | Ductal carcinoma in situ |
| DDx: | Differential diagnosis |

| | |
|---|---|
| DIC: | Disseminated intravascular coagulation |
| DM: | Diabetes mellitus |
| DNI: | Do not intubate |
| DNR: | Do not resuscitate |
| DOA: | Dead on arrival |
| DOB: | Date of birth |
| DOC: | Drug of choice |
| DOE: | Dyspnea on exertion |
| DP: | Dorsalis pedis pulse |
| DPL: | Diagnostic peritoneal lavage |
| DUI : | Driving under the influence—intoxicated |
| DVT: | Deep vein thrombosis |
| Dx: | Diagnosis |
| | |
| ECASA: | Enteric-coated ASA (aspirin) |
| ECG: | Electrocardiogram |
| EENT: | Eyes, Ears, Nose, and Throat |
| EGD: | Endoscopic gastroduodenoscopy |
| ENT: | Ear, nose, throat (otolaryngologist) |
| ERCP: | Endoscopic retrograde cholangiopancreatography |
| ESRD: | End-stage renal disease |
| EtOH: | Ethanol or Ethyl alcohol |
| ETT: | Endotracheal tube |
| | |
| f/u: | Follow-up |
| FBS: | Fasting blood sugar |
| Fe: | Iron |
| FH: | Family history |
| FSP: | Fibrin split products |
| FSBG or FSBS: | Finger stick blood glucose/sugar |
| FTA: | Fluorescent treponemal antibody absorption |
| FTI: | Free thyroxin index |
| FTT: | Failure to thrive |
| FUO: | Fever of unknown origin |
| Fx: | Fracture |
| | |
| G5P4013: | Gravida 5 Para 4014 = 5 pregnancies, 4 term deliveries, 0 stillbirths, 1 abortion, 4 live births |
| GCS: | Glasgow Coma Scale |

271

| | |
|---|---|
| GFR: | Glomerular filtratration rate |
| GH: | Growth hormone |
| GI: | Gastrointestinal |
| GSW: | Gunshot wound |
| GT: | Gastrostomy tube |
| gtt: | "Guttae," drops |
| GTT: | Glucose tolerance test |
| GU: | Genitourinary |
| | |
| h/o: | History of |
| H&P: | History and physical |
| HA: | Headache |
| HAL or | |
| HyperAl: | Hyperalimentation |
| HCO$_3$: | Bicarbonate |
| Hct: | Hematocrit |
| HCTZ: | Hydrochlorothiazide |
| HEENT: | Head, Eyes, Ears, Nose, and Throat |
| Heplock: | Heparin lock |
| HO: | House officer |
| HOB: | Head of bed |
| HPI: | History of present illness |
| HRRR: | Heart regular rate and rhythm |
| HTN: | Hypertension |
| Hx: | History |
| | |
| I&Os: | Ins and Outs |
| ICP: | Intracranial pressure |
| ICU: | Intensive care unit |
| IDDM: | Insulin-dependent diabetes mellitus |
| IM: | Intramuscular |
| IV: | Intravenous, or intravenous line |
| IVDA: | IV drug abuse |
| IVP: | Intravenous pyelogram |
| | |
| JVD: | Jugular venous distention |
| | |
| LLE: | Left lower extremity |
| LCTA: | Lungs clear to auscultation |

| | |
|---|---|
| LE: | Lower extremities |
| LGIB: | Lower gastrointestinal bleeding |
| LLL: | Left lower lobe |
| LOC: | Loss of consciousness |
| LR: | Lactated Ringer's IV solution |
| LVEDP: | Left ventricular end diastolic pressure |
| | |
| MDI: | Metered-dose inhaler (with or w/o spacer) |
| $MgSO_4$: | Magnesium sulfate |
| MI: | Myocardial infarction |
| MOM: | Milk of magnesia |
| MR: | Mitral regurgitation |
| MRG: | Murmurs, rubs, gallops—m/r/g |
| MS: | Morphine sulfate |
| MVA: | Motor vehicle accident |
| | |
| N/V/D/C: | Nausea/vomiting/diarrhea/constipation |
| NAD: | No acute distress or No apparent distress |
| NC: | Nasal cannula |
| NC/AT: | Normocephalic/atraumatic |
| ND: | Nondistended |
| NG or NGT: | Nasogastric tube |
| NKDA: | No known drug allergies |
| Nl: | Normal |
| NPH: | Normal pressure hydrocephalus |
| NPH: | Neutral protamine Hagedorn (intermediate-acting insulin) |
| NPO: | Nil per os (nothing by mouth) |
| NS: | Normal saline (0.9% NaCl) |
| NSAID: | Nonsteriodal antiinflammatory drug |
| NSR: | Normal sinus rhythm |
| NT: | Nontender |
| NT/ND: | Nontender/Nondistended |
| NTG: | Nitroglycerin |
| | |
| $O_2$: | Oxygen |
| OC: | Oral contraceptive |
| OCTOR: | On call to OR |
| OD: | Overdose |

| | |
|---|---|
| OOB: | Out of bed (to chair) |
| OT: | Occupational therapy |
| | |
| p: | Pending |
| P&PD: | Percussion and postural drainage |
| PAC: | Premature atrial contraction |
| PAT: | Paroxysmal atrial tachycardia |
| PCA: | Patient-controlled analgesia |
| PCN: | Penicillin |
| PCP: | *Pneumocystis carinii* pneumonia |
| PCr: | Plasma creatinine |
| PCWP: | Pulmonary capillary wedge pressure |
| pCXR: | Portable chest x-ray |
| PDA: | Patent ductus arteriosus |
| PE: | Pulmonary embolus |
| PEA: | Pulseless electrical activity |
| PEEP: | Positive end expiratory pressure |
| PEG: | Percutaneous endoscopic gastrostomy (gastric tube) |
| PERRL: | Pupils equally round and reactive to light |
| PERRLA: | Pupils equally round and reactive to light and accommodation |
| PET: | Positron emission tomography |
| PID: | Pelvic inflammatory disease |
| PND: | Paroxysmal nocturnal dyspnea |
| PO: | Per os (by mouth) |
| ppd: | cigarette packs per day |
| PPD: | Protein purified derivative (tuberculosis skin test) |
| PRN: | Pro re nata (as the need arises) |
| PSA: | Prostate specific antigen |
| PSVT: | Paroxysmal supraventricular tachycardia |
| Pt: | Patient |
| PT: | Physical therapy; Prothrombin time |
| PTC: | Percutaneous transhepatic cholangiogram |
| PTCA: | Percutaneous transluminal coronary angioplasty |
| PTT: | Partial thromboplastin time |
| PTX: | Pneumothorax |
| PVC: | Premature ventricular contraction |

| | |
|---|---|
| q8h: | Taken every 8 hours |
| qd: | Each day |
| qhs: | At bedtime |
| qid: | Quarter in die ($4 \times$ daily) |
| | |
| RUE: | Right upper extremity |
| RUQ: | Right upper quadrant |
| RBBB: | Right bundle branch block |
| RLL: | Right lower lobe |
| r/o: | Rule out |
| ROS: | Review of systems |
| Roux-en-Y: | Gastrojejunostomy and duodenojejunostomy |
| RR: | Respiratory rate |
| RRR: | Regular rate and rhythm |
| RUL: | Right upper lobe |
| Rx: | Prescription |
| | |
| $SaO_2$: | $O_2$ saturation |
| SBP: | Systolic blood pressure |
| SCDs: | Sequential compression devices |
| SDP: | Single donor platelets |
| SEM: | Systolic ejection murmur |
| SOAP: | Progress note: Subjective, Objective, Assessment, and Plan |
| SOB: | Shortness of breath (dyspnea) |
| s/p: | Status post (e.g., status after an event, procedure) |
| SQ: | Subcutaneous |
| Std: | Standard |
| STD: | Sexually transmitted disease |
| SVT: | Supraventricular tachycardia |
| Sx: | Symptoms |
| | |
| TAH/BSO: | Total abdominal hysterectomy/bilateral salpingo-oophorectomy |
| TB: | Tuberculosis |
| TBI: | Traumatic brain injury |
| T&C: | Type and cross |
| TC&DB: | Turn, cough, and deep breathe |

| | |
|---|---|
| TEE: | Transesophageal echocardiogram |
| TIA: | Transient ischemic attack |
| tid: | Three times per day |
| TKO: | To keep open |
| TPA: | Tissue plasminogen activator |
| TPN: | Total parenteral nutrition |
| TURP: | Transurethral resection of prostate |
| TV: | Tidal volume |
| Tx: | Treatment |
| | |
| U: | Unit |
| UA: | Urine analysis |
| UGIB: | Upper gastrointestinal bleeding |
| U/P: | Urine/plasma ratio |
| URI: | Upper respiratory infection |
| ut dict: | From "ut dictum," as directed |
| US: | Ultrasound |
| UTI: | Urinary tract infection |
| | |
| VF: | Ventricular fibrillation |
| VQ: | Ventilation/perfusion, V/Q scan |
| VS: | Vital sign |
| VT: | Ventricular tachycardia |
| | |
| w/: | With |
| w/o: | Without |
| WBC: | White blood cell |
| WD: | Wet to dry dressing |
| WDWN: | Well-developed, well-nourished |
| WNL or wnl: | Within normal limits |
| | |
| y/o: | Years old |

# Index

Page numbers followed by *f* refer to figures; those followed by *t* refer to tables.